Mind Body Kitchen

A Loving Approach to Set Yourself Free

Lindsey Antman

Mind Body Kitchen

A Loving Approach to Set Yourself Free

The information contained in this book is based on the life experiences and opinions perceived and expressed by the author.

Published, distributed, and printed in the United States of America by Rose Gold Publishing, LLC.

ISBN: 978-1-952070-39-6

www.RoseGoldPublishingLLC.com

Table of Contents

Chapters

Dedication

This book is dedicated to anyone who has ever felt stuck, frustrated, or conflicted by the pressures and demands of the modern world. Trust your gut, my friend.

For my children, the beautiful beings I would be grateful to have and raise one day, I hope that by the time you read these words, body neutrality and heart-centered, holistic wellness practices have already become normalized in your world. I hope that the inner battles I write about in these pages don't make any sense because they don't apply to you. I love you, and you are perfect, just the way you are.

Acknowledgement

I wish I knew how to thank every person who has ever directly or indirectly impacted the coach, the teacher, the student, the partner, the lover, the friend, the human I am today. To each individual who, consciously or unconsciously, has shared their experience and wisdom with me, thank you!

To my parents, thank you for everything. One million ways to say I love you would still not be enough to express how much you mean to me. The relationship we have is so rare and amazing; I'm learning how to not take that for granted. You already know the infinite ways in which you deserve so much love and thanks, but just so everyone here reading this knows, my beautiful, respectable, supportive, encouraging, kind, and devoted parents have had the most significant influence on who I am. They are my rock and my reason for wanting to become the best version of myself.

To my partner, Jeremy, you are amazing, and you deserve just as much credit and appreciation. You've made a profound impact on my motivation and my drive over the years, as well as my ability to build a business and write a book at this stage of my life. Thank you for your support, your guidance, your kindness, and your belief in me. You've seen my potential in the moments I didn't see it. You've held me in the moments I didn't know how to embrace myself. I love you and appreciate you more than you'll ever know. Thank you for being in my life.

To one of my yoga mentors, who I am grateful to call my first, Jill. I often reflect on the journey of life, how one event leads to another, and how every decision we make impacts the direction of our story. I remember how we met when I decided to take on a part-time position at the studio you were managing. Timing is everything, and I'll never forget the morning you encouraged me to sign up for the Yoga Sculpt teacher training… You could have easily not said anything about it, especially since the training was starting only one week from that day! But you saw something in me that I didn't see in myself. – a yoga teacher. I filled out the form and made the deposit that day, mostly because I was so excited to learn from you!

My yoga practice, my career, and my life have all been enhanced and more fulfilled since becoming a yoga teacher… and I have YOU to thank for that.

Thank you, Jill, for the guidance you give, the presence you create, and the wisdom you share in each and every class. You are a light!

To the Institute for the Psychology of Eating, thank you for existing. To Marc David, the Founder, thank you for having the curiosity and the courage to go where very few practitioners in your field were willing to or able to explore - a more heart-centered and real approach to healing through nutrition and psychology. During my undergrad, while studying Nutrition and Dietetics, I was intentionally taught that addressing the necessary areas of wellness and healing, such as thoughts, feelings, emotions, spirituality, sexuality, social well-being, etc., were not ethical for us as "nutritionists" to talk about with our clients. How could anyone possibly believe that food and diet *alone* can heal? I realize now, through discovering your program, how impactful and essential the approach you teach can be for many individuals and communities. When I found your coaching certification program, my eyes lit up. I simply searched "mind-body nutrition" out of curiosity and intuition, and there you were! Right there before me with everything I knew in my heart and deep in my gut but didn't yet have the tools or language to put into practice. I would not be where I am personally or professionally without this program that has brought so much insight into my own battles with food and body image, that I was not previously aware of. Thank you for guiding my own healing and for permitting me to coach others in such a meaningful and transformational way.

To my writing coach, publisher, and good friend, Dolly Cortes, thank you! Writing this book would not have been possible without you.

Introduction

We are all perfectly imperfect, and that is what makes you, me, us, beautiful. You are enough.

Once you choose to accept and embrace yourself fully, you hold the power to master your thoughts, find beauty in the chaos, and create the life you desire. Once you decide to love yourself unconditionally, you discover the guidance you need to find peace from all the head noise and overwhelm in your mind, experience how it feels to be at home in your body, learn how to tap into and trust your intuition.

Why this book? Why now?

I see you; I get you; I empathize with you. This book was inspired by an emotional breakdown at 2:00 AM one Saturday morning, which you'll hear more about in this book. I am not perfect, but I have come a tremendously long way on my personal journey towards self-love, patience, acceptance, and choosing to live my truth.

For that and so much more, I am proud. My passion now is guiding and teaching others how to incorporate the skills I've learned - as a certified eating psychology coach, yoga teacher, and student of life - through my coaching company, Mind Body Kitchen.

My motivation to write is to make sure that women who feel alone in their thoughts and are unhappy in their body, who are struggling to figure it all out with food and reach their wellness goals, will feel noticed and understood when they get to know me. This book is for the woman who, on the outside, has everything going for her, yet wonders why she still doesn't feel completely fulfilled or at ease. This is the book you pick up to remind yourself *you are not alone*. From personal experience, that feeling, that knowing, in itself has so much power to heal.

Whatever you're facing now - any amount of stress, anxiety, overthinking, overwhelm, feeling of being out of control or the fear of not being good enough - you don't have to face it alone or in silence. By sharing some of my story and the stories of other women, I hope to make a positive difference by reminding you that you *do* have a voice and it matters. YOU matter. Whenever you feel lost or misunderstood, trapped in fear and self-doubt…Turn to this book for a reminder that you are enough as you are in this moment, and in each moment as it comes.

Say it with me… "I AM ENOUGH."

Too much of the modern world makes us believe we are never good enough, smart enough, pretty enough, sexy enough, skinny enough, healthy enough, strong enough, successful enough, talented enough, worthy enough… When will we allow ourselves to be okay with who we are and where we are at this moment on our unique journey?

It's quite a challenge, I believe, to be surrounded by a culture that is powered by billions of dollars in marketing and advertising by companies whose intentions are to make us feel, at our core, not enough…

So, we buy more, search for more, and without even knowing, we risk being entirely controlled, being led towards the next best thing… the next 'right' thing… got to have it… and if we don't? We think we're falling short.

These messages travel from the outside world and penetrate our soul, consuming our every thought and every choice we make. I'll share some of the ways I've struggled with this kind of conditioning that once affected the relationships I had with my body, with food, with my thoughts, with my health, and even with other people.

What grounds me and makes me feel more "okay" are the moments when I realize I'm not alone - that other people are going through or have been through similar experiences. And it reminds me, over and over, that when we speak our truth, we induce hope and reason for other humans to speak and follow *their* truth. By holding back out of fear of what others might think of us, we stay stuck and alone and exacerbate the problems that our silence creates. So, I choose to speak up, even if other people see me differently because of it.

The truth is, we all go through tough things - that's the beautiful chaos of being human. We need each other, and we also need to learn how to look within, get comfortable with being who we truly are and where we are; trust ourselves and our intuition, and love ourselves completely, wholeheartedly, without conditions.

Only you can guarantee your own happiness, and that might sound like a challenge on its own if you don't unconditionally love and accept yourself. By choosing to read a book like this one, I'm confident you're already on a path worth taking in this world - one that seeks true love from Self over acceptance from others. I hope that by the end of this book, you will have a greater sense of confidence to walk through life being more aware, more awake, more alive on your journey of well-being.

This book gives you unconditional permission to listen to your inner wisdom as you learn what it takes to come back to yourself for guidance whenever you feel unsure of which direction to go in. There is so much freedom in deeply listening to and honoring your gut feelings as you embrace the power of trusting yourself over perfecting yourself. Only self-love can take you to where you desperately want to arrive. Ready or not, turn the page. Let's do this together!

Chapter 1

One Question

On a Friday night, in November 2020, I kissed my partner on the cheek, said goodnight, and I asked him what time he planned on coming to bed. He replied, "Soon, about 30 minutes." He meant it; I know it. But he has this funny habit of falling asleep on the couch.

I remember lying in bed slightly cold (he's my human heater), and I couldn't wait for him to join me and hold me tight. But I sort of went to sleep with the feeling that he might not make it from the couch to the bed… again. He had been working incredibly long and draining hours at work. We were both aware of the two weeks that he would be pretty much unavailable at home, but I'm not sure if I was entirely prepared for how that would affect me emotionally during that time.

I used to struggle with insomnia. My partner can fall asleep literally anywhere at any time, which I could never understand because I can only fall asleep in a dark room with my own space in just the right temperature, eye mask on and earplugs in; silence and total peace. I have my ways of winding down at night to get myself "ready" for bed. For me, falling asleep on the couch during a movie or with a bunch of people around would rarely happen. Right now, my routine looks like stretching, meditating, drinking herbal tea, taking my valerian root supplement, washing up and I'm (hopefully) ready for a good night's sleep. My man likes to call me a High Maintenance Sleeper. It's true! While that's me, he on the other hand can sleep like a baby while sitting upright on an airplane with turbulence!

His ability to fall asleep so easily and comfortably was always something that I was jealous of. I would feel increasingly frustrated anytime I was battling my insomnia because I would just think, damn, he makes it look so easy! He later told me it wasn't always that way for him, that he had to work on this for a long time and find his little tricks to relax his mind and body for quality sleep, anywhere, any time. But still… my own insecurity, frustration and comparison gets the best of me at times.

So, there's a little backstory for you. A quality night's sleep is crucial for me to function because I can be an emotional wreck without it. And on that particular Friday night in November, my good night's sleep was ruined… *by my own relentless thoughts.*

I fell asleep around 10 p.m. and slept great for a few hours. When I woke up around 2 a.m., the moonlight was softly shining into the bedroom. I glanced over to see the blanket still perfectly made on his side of the bed. In that very instant, my brain was fully charged, powered on with emotion; I shot up out of bed and stomped into the living room to find him cozied up in the corner of the couch. This really shouldn't have been a big deal to me… I knew he just fell asleep and all I had to do was ask him to come to bed, which I did… But in the minutes that followed, as we made our way to the bedroom, I noticed myself getting gradually heated and upset. I wasn't entirely sure why.

I tried to go back to bed but I couldn't. All I could think about was that he would probably fall fast asleep in bed in a matter of seconds like nothing happened, like he didn't just sleep for three hours on the couch without realizing he wasn't next to me… And here I am, wide awake! *Why didn't he just come to bed? He told me he would... So, what the hell?* That was only the trigger. What happened next most certainly had nothing to do with him falling asleep on the couch or our relationship in general.

My mind started racing, going off in all different directions. I can't even remember all the places my mind traveled, but it was enough to know that I would most likely be tossing and turning for a while if I stayed in bed, so I decided to go to the living room to meditate, breathe, and quiet my thoughts before going back to bed. All I remember happening next was that I could feel the pressure building in my head, the tears started swelling, the lump in my throat was hardening, and I realized… Oh crap, here it comes… I'm about to have a meltdown in the middle of the night. This has happened before, so I felt it coming, and I think a part of me was okay with letting it happen… Emotions are meant to be felt, not denied.

Therapy taught me that if I need to cry, I should give myself permission to let it out, unleash the feeling, release the tension. But this… this was too much. I was sweating, shivering, shaking and sobbing about absolutely nothing and everything simultaneously!

Mind you, it’s 2020. We're coming to the end of a year when the world is facing a global pandemic: Anxiety, stress, fatigue, uncertainty, and over-whelmed feelings, are what most of the population is looking at daily. So, I wasn't alone and was very aware of the circumstances. But just because these feelings were expected to arise doesn't make them any easier to deal with.

So, there I was, sitting on the couch, swaddled in a fuzzy blanket, sitting pretzel style, feeling small and crying in the dark with only the moonlight filling the space around me. By the way, I was still wearing my earplugs at this point, so the stillness of silence made my thoughts seem even louder. After about half an hour of being there on the couch all alone, less than 30 feet from the bedroom where my partner was asleep, my thoughts went in a new direction. *How has he not heard me yet?? Why hasn't he come out here to check if I'm okay??? I'm sure he is sleeping soundly... He doesn't even know. Damn it, why do I have to be the one who is a light sleeper?! He can sleep through anything with his stupid selective hearing, drown out anything, even my pain.*

I couldn't sit with the loneliness anymore, so I yanked out my earplugs, and at the height of my panic attack, with tears streaming down my face, I screamed, "Can you just fucking come out here, please???" Just. Like. That.

He got up. Completely out of it from sleep, but he did.

This man loves me so much, and I love him. But even then, as he snuggled up next to me, I felt even more alone as I stayed put in my own head, still trying to decipher my thoughts… What the heck is this all about? It hurt my heart so bad I just wanted to close my eyes and escape the discomfort. I wanted to erase the night and pretend it never happened, wishing at this point that I had just stayed in bed and left him on the couch. This wasn't how I wanted my partner to see me, either. But he cares for me and would do anything for me.

As a human being on planet Earth, this wasn't my first emotional breakdown, and I don't expect it to be the last one in my lifetime. As it was happening, I knew I'd be just fine the next day and feel completely different about myself and my life - thinking about the good and positive things. But at the moment, I didn't know what to do! Using self-awareness to recognize my thoughts but not react to them is a lifelong practice... These overwhelming thoughts don't magically go away. You just get better and better at responding to them with love and kindness rather than reacting to them with shame and doubt.

Our thoughts can be so powerful, sometimes to the point of literally consuming us from the inside out. With mindfulness, we can take back our control. We don't have to let our thoughts claim any power over us, but during that hour, I let my thoughts take the reins. I let them run wild, and I take full responsibility for that.

After sitting on the couch with him, I was starting to feel completely defeated and was getting so sick of listening to these thoughts. I was more than ready just to give it a rest and surrender - to go to bed and close my eyes, even if I were to lay awake with my thoughts for the rest of the night. Then something I wasn't expecting happened. The air around me fell still when he finally interrupted my unproductive, internal tantrum by asking me one question.

It ended up being the most important question of the night - far above my dozens of fear-based, self-doubting ideas that consumed me for nearly an hour.

In the most casual and calm voice, he asked me, "*Do you love yourself*?"

Chapter 2

The Truth

So, who am I and why did I decide to write this book? First impressions *are* important, so you might be wondering why I started this book on that particular note - sharing a story about a meltdown I had one night? Well, although that story may not be the best portrayal of who I am, it's the reason you're reading this book. Okay, maybe not the *only* reason, but it was the finger that pulled the trigger on YEARS of thinking about it. I've listened to friends, colleagues, clients and family members tell me how much they enjoy my writing and that I should write a book. There were many times I questioned my voice or felt unsure of what I would write about. On that early Saturday morning, in the moments after

I picked myself back up, exhausted from the tears and lack of sleep, I realized how much I DO love myself. But I am human. We are all beautifully, imperfectly, mysteriously, human.

It's time we make loving ourselves a non-negotiable priority. This is something that I know from experience takes time and patience as you transform your wellness journey into a more positive one - a less analytical, less critical, less judgmental experience. Loving and accepting yourself may not feel entirely easy the very moment that you decide to, but it does start with a *decision.*

Self-love is a constant choice. Even after years of putting my own well-being and happiness first so that everything else could naturally fall into place, I still have my moments where I'm not totally content with what's going on in my head or how I feel about where I am on my journey. When I discover new parts of myself that I want to change or improve, I can be especially hard on myself. Let's be real, we're all our own worst critics! But that's just the challenge… We are constantly evolving, learning and growing. If we've stopped learning new information about ourselves, we've stopped being curious, or we just aren't aware anymore. Don't trip yourself up and believe you'll find this magical place of self-love and never have doubts or fears or negative thoughts ever again… It takes conscious, daily effort to choose self-love; and believing in yourself no matter what you've been through certainly takes a courageous amount of effort and self-acceptance.

But it's not impossible. Once you decide that loving yourself *matters* for your health and well-being, it becomes easier over time. When you love yourself better, you'll know how to take care of yourself better. And even better, when you know how to love yourself, you can tap into the power of truly loving others. It all starts with a decision. Every day is a new day to start again. So, start right now. Decide to work on loving and accepting yourself, *all parts of yourself* - on the good days *and* on the bad days.

EVERY PART OF YOU is worth loving.

So around 3:00 AM on that whirlwind of a Saturday morning, I had this thought... *I know I'm not alone in feeling alone.* I could only imagine that everyone has those moments from time to time. I essentially wrote this book as a reminder that you are not alone and that you are enough as you are today. So never for one second doubt who you are or how far you've come on your journey.

Whether I'm talking to a yoga student or a fellow teacher, a coaching client or a colleague, a good friend or someone I just met, my intent is to listen.

Stories are so powerful, and I'm always fascinated and eager to learn from another person's journey. I recognize I am not perfect (no one is), nor do I have all the answers in life (no one does) … So, I always do my best to meet another person where they are, connect with their story, and walk *with* them towards the next best step on their journey. We're all here in life trying to make sense of it all, and no one should ever feel alone or less, no matter what happens.

Before writing this chapter, I realized that I was nominated for the spotlight sister of the month in a women's networking organization I'm a part of. One of my sisters wrote, *"Lindsey has a heart for entrepreneurship and growth as a person. She is generous with her time, an incredible teacher, and has a good spirit. And her belief that people are capable of change is nothing short of inspirational."*

I read that and I honestly teared up a little. I felt that warm, fuzzy feeling of gratitude, and it only made me want to give so much more! It warms my heart when I hear positive and encouraging feedback from other women, especially those I admire for their work ethic, wisdom, good heart, and authenticity. When people say nice things about me, I enjoy it, but not because I rely on that reassurance or validation to get ahead… I know the value I bring to the table. However, I used the thrive (in the short term) on any confirmation I could get from others that I was enough; but still, I hardly believed it in my core. Now I know better and have done the inner work to prove it to myself.

Hearing these heartfelt words makes me feel good today because they reflect how I am showing up in the world, which is important to me. I am doing my best to make a positive difference, even if I can brighten one person's day each day, that is enough.

My personal and professional mission is to remind people how much they matter, because let's be honest, all women want to feel important and appreciated. They also want to be seen and understood. They want to feel certain that their voice is heard and that their message has been received. So, the message that my friend wrote when nominating me as the spotlight sister of the month was a totally unexpected and genuine confirmation of that for me.

Last week I even had two different people privately message me, sharing the same exact thing. With it, they said, "Hey, this reminded me of you."

It was a shared post that a woman wrote about her daughter, who had expressed love and acceptance towards her own changing body. The message behind it was that if everyone possessed her level of body confidence, then the diet industry would fail. I loved that! It was another reminder that people are hearing my message as an eating psychology coach and that my brand is gaining awareness. It feels amazing to know that when people hear about mindful eating, self-love, or the importance of questioning our diet-crazy culture, they think of me. It took me almost two years of consistent effort to get any real momentum in my business and create powerful messaging that is now being reflected to me. I used to be the girl who often felt misunderstood and entitled to be liked by everyone. Today I am a woman who says what needs to be said, remains as kind and as humble as possible, and is not afraid to go against the grain to make a point or share what I feel in my heart and know in my gut.

One thing I am certain of is that I do not give up. I may be hard on myself at times, but I always make it through and eventually look back on what once seemed like the hardest thing I had ever faced and think, what was I so worried about? I have conquered many obstacles in my life, and I am stronger because of them, but that doesn't minimize the challenges or take away any part of my personal experience. The whole reason I am writing this book is to remind you that you will overcome whatever is holding you back, that you are stronger than you'll ever know and that one day you'll appreciate the lessons you've learned because of your experiences. But where you are now is perfectly okay. You are not alone. We all have our dull moments. We need the darkness to appreciate the light.

Deciding to start a business from scratch by myself at 24 years old was a huge challenge. It was a positive change, for sure, but it wasn't all "I get to work from home in my PJs now and take long walks while deciding how much money I want to make this year," which is how it can sometimes look from the outside while scrolling through #bossbabes on social media.

Building a business is hard work. It's scary, unpredictable, and it means that whatever personal development I was doing before I was self-employed had to be tripled! I wonder about quitting sometimes and think how much easier it would be to just work for someone else and get a consistent paycheck. If that's you, no shame! Good for you! Everyone must choose what fulfills *their* hearts, and I realized that doing a job that didn't fulfill me or challenge me was not enough. I tried it, hated it, and moved on. Even better, at this point in my career, as my business coach likes to phrase it, I'm "basically unemployable." I can be way too independent and stubborn at times. I can get flustered in stressful environments, especially when I'm having a hard day and need more time and space to recharge. I can't tell you how many times I hid away in a bathroom, in the stairwell, or in a friend's office during my last corporate job. If my old boss is reading this, sorry for that.

But being your own boss isn't necessarily easier. At first, I thought having a flexible schedule, working when, how, and with whom I wanted would be the ultimate dream. I quickly realized that having this kind of freedom is really hard, creating new obstacles to work through! It also forces me to look closely at myself in order to discover my own desires and boundaries. I have put so much time and energy into my own personal growth over the last few years, and it shows by who I am today. For that, I am grateful.

Whether you are your own boss or not, whether you work or not, take time to step back and appreciate your journey. Acknowledge all the obstacles you've overcome to get to where you are today! Explore all the ways in which you are a better version of yourself because of all you've been through.

I can share that I am strong, open-minded, curious, smart, kind, empathetic, honest, and I'm not afraid to speak my mind, even when there's a lump in my throat. When I feel unsure, I take the next best step forward anyway. When I stand up to share my story and I'm so nervous I can't feel my face, I shine my big, happy, energizing smile and hope they don't notice I'm trying not to pee in my pants. When I'm questioning who I am, I take a deep breath, look within, and remind myself of exactly who I am!

I saw a movie once and heard the cutest line, "If your

hands are shaking, turn them into jazz hands." That's what I aim for every day. It's not about faking it… You don't need to fake anything to be successful because you already are successful. When I guide my students, I remind them that they are amazing too, just as they are, and they have already accomplished so much in their life to feel proud of. Oftentimes the root of our own unhappiness and inability to acknowledge our success, feeling that we're never good enough, is rooted in our own comparison and the false belief that we need to be like everyone else if we want to succeed in the world.

Comparison used to affect me deep in my core. I compared my body, my eating habits, my intelligence, my dance moves, my sex life, my relationships, my bank account, and even my outward confidence. I have learned to practice letting go of comparing myself to other people, which has taken me so very far. When I show up as my authentic self and choose to be ME, there is no one I could ever compare myself to. I am the only me. I may not always know the words to express it, but I feel it. I know who I've been and who I am today. I'm even more excited and open to discovering who I am becoming. Each day is a chance to feel for what I want and what makes me happy, and that is what I hope you can discover too.

You are you, and that is perfect.

Take some time to journal now

- *Write the beautiful truth about YOU.*
- *Which positive qualities would your family, friends, or partner share about you?*
- *How does God, the Universe, a higher power, or whatever you believe in, see you?*

It's fine (and sometimes healthy) to brag about yourself a little! Go for it!

Chapter 3

Rose-Colored Glasses

It's the middle of December, the year which we all collectively faced and endured a global pandemic. We're still in it, and on top of that, it's cold and dark. I thrive in the warmth and natural light of our Midwest sunshine, so when the days get shorter, and the weather gets frigid, I just want to hibernate! I used to brush this off as the winter blues, but I'm learning now that this is a very real, biological challenge that millions of people experience each year when the seasons change. This year has been especially challenging for me to manage, so I make a daily commitment to love and respect my body no matter what - to surrender.

I found myself pacing around my house one morning, not sure what to do with myself… Again, being my own boss, sometimes I get too much time on my hands and too much space to think! Today I felt like calling the whole thing off, pressing pause. I don't want to keep trying to be perfect and optimistic all the time… It really is exhausting! Lately, I've been noticing how much harder it's getting to write, to set goals, to inspire, to uplift other people, to be a leader, and to be a healer… When I am still doing my own inner work.

It takes a lot of energy to put yourself out there, to do something you've never done, and wanting to do a good job at it while simultaneously surrendering to knowing your work is not perfect. Finding that balance is tough, coming from a person who has a history of striving for perfection - it's something I am constantly learning and relearning to let go of. I realized today that part of the reason I could be sabotaging myself from stepping up is that I'm worried about my performance under the circumstances. Thoughts keep swirling around in my head…

I'm not in the right state of mind to do this today.

I'll just wait until I'm feeling better.

Who am I to help other people when I can barely get myself out of bed?

But I know deep down that none of that really matters, and it's actually not even true. I don't need to be perfect to do a good job. I'm learning through my own self-awareness. There will be good days and bad days, beautiful moments as well as some pretty ugly moments. The greatest question that Life asks us each and every day is this ***"Are you willing to show up, fully and authentically, in the best way that you possibly can with what you have, today?"***

Not tomorrow when things are better. Not at some point in the future when things get easier. Because that is never a guarantee.

I hear this kind of thing all the time from the women I talk to. Some people will literally put their lives on hold as if they can't go after what they want until something else is fixed first. I refer to it as the "I'll be *this* when *that*" dilemma.

I'll be successful when I make over $100,000

I'll be sexy when I can finally fit into that one dress at that particular store

I'll be healthy when I can finally stop binge eating

I'll be worthy of love and affection when every ounce of fat around my midsection is gone

I'll be happy when I lose this weight

I'll be healed when I no longer have negative

thoughts

Who says you're not already successful, sexy, healthy, worthy of love, worthy of happiness, or healed? You have the power and the ability to be all of those things right now! Don't believe me? It's because you are choosing to believe differently - it's all about what you focus on. What you think, you become.

What I see happening with the "I'll be this when that" dilemma is that we are setting unrealistic and unfair expectations on ourselves, oftentimes without consciously realizing we are doing it. We decide that the only way to get the thing we want should be based on specific measures of success.

When we get too caught up in our own imaginary cause-and-effect scenarios, we miss out on all the possibilities and opportunities for success that may come our way… Ones which allow us to have or create what we want *right now*, in this very season of our lives!

Using myself as an example, I was stuck in my writing because of my own conditions I put on myself. I believed something along the lines of, "I'll be more qualified to make a difference when I get my shit together." Really?? If everyone believed that was true, then there would be no more leaders in the world - no more teachers or guides or mentors or coaches. None of us have all our stuff figured out! And anyone who tries to tell you they do is full of crap. Admittedly, the fact that I *don't* have everything 'figured out' is what makes me so good at what I do. I choose to walk alongside my clients' journey, to feel with them and to be with them, not to know it all and pretend I have more authority than they do.

Coaches are constantly learning and growing, themselves. The truth is that I don't have to be perfect to share from my perspective, and neither do you. One of my mentors helped me realize this when he shared that coaches are often drawn towards teaching the things they still need to learn as well. It makes sense! The specific topics we care the most about are usually the ones which reflect our own personal journeys. The greatest thought leaders don't teach from textbooks; they share wisdom using stories, speak from their hearts, and reflect on their own life experiences. I don't have all the answers, and I still remind myself from time to time that it's *okay* to not know all the answers.

This morning, during a conversation about a text message that my partner and I perceived slightly differently... I was trying to explain my point, and he told me I was putting on rose-colored glasses. At first, I had no idea what he was talking about. He told me I was looking for optimism in a situation that didn't necessarily require my positive twist because there was nothing wrong with it in the first place. In his eyes, I saw the situation from a negative point of view, and I was distorting reality. At that moment, I was actually sabotaging my own happiness based on what I saw. I was looking to change the perspective when perhaps there really was nothing to change! When he responded with, "That's a negative way of looking at it," my immediate reaction was anger and defensiveness because I thought, "Hold on, no! I'm not a negative person!" But that's not even what he meant. And it didn't hit me until now as I write this story… What he was trying to say was that the world isn't perfect, but it's not all bad.

People aren't perfect. I'm not perfect… and it's fine.

He was absolutely right about my own self-sabotage at that moment. I don't have to put on my rose-colored glasses every time I don't like what I see, whether it's something in my external reality - what's happening around me - or something about my internal reality - my own imperfection. Sometimes we don't see things in the best light or from the most positive lens, and that's okay! It doesn't necessarily make you a nasty, negative person. But here is another opportunity to practice self-awareness and to get curious with yourself.

How do I see this and WHY don't I like what I see?

What is triggering my desire to change the situation or control how other people see it?

Am I willing to remain open to criticism and feedback without getting defensive when someone else doesn't share my point of view?

How does what I see in the world reflect what I see in myself?

Rose-colored glasses work in two ways.

Sometimes we seek to change our perspective of the world by clouding the negative to only see the positive. Don't get me wrong; this can be totally necessary! I'm notorious for it... But if we do this all the time, we may forget the downside of constantly wearing these super cool spectacles - we risk clouding our view of our internal reality as well. We avoid seeing the hard parts of ourselves - the stuff we would rather not acknowledge or deal with. However, that in itself is a form of self-sabotage.

There is so much we can do to improve the world around us by looking at the things that make us uncomfortable, a global pandemic, global warming, hunger, homelessness, or domestic violence, for example. We MUST look at these things if we wish to improve them. If we want to grow personally, from the inside out, then the same rule applies. It's impossible to grow if we refuse to look at our own shadows, right in the face, unclouded, uncolored.

Put on your clear, magnifying glasses, my friends! It's no mystery that life is a mystery. We won't always get it right or have a perfect view of the world, and that's okay. But as we open our hearts to learn about the world - the beautiful and the chaotic parts - we must also choose to learn about ourselves - ALL of ourselves - and that takes a tremendous amount of courage.

Later today, after a great virtual yoga session with a client, followed by a networking call, I noticed the sun was really coming through the clouds and onto my patio. I'm super sensitive to the cold and I can be a real baby about it. But I chose to put my big girl panties on (and a sweater and a jacket) to catch a few minutes of rays on my face and breathe some fresh air into my lungs. I wore my sunglasses and imagined I was lounging on the beach. This morning, as the sun was still hiding behind the clouds and just barely peeking out to brighten this cold December day, getting out of bed was a challenge... So, for me, getting outside was a big deal.

It won't always be easy to walk through your journey, so remember to be kind to yourself. As you learn to notice and listen to your thoughts, as you learn to acknowledge and honor what your body tells you, remember to love yourself through it all. Because doing the things that seem even the most obvious (like going outside or exercising or eating healthy) can be really hard sometimes! Celebrate all the tiny wins. Seriously, every small step counts.

You can choose to put your rose-colored glasses on to avoid the sucky stuff when it's just too damn hard to acknowledge the truth. Use them to help you get through the hard days if it makes the world seem a little less scary. But remember to whip out your magnifying glasses from time to time…

Look at your TRUTH so you can LEARN and GROW from it. You are so brave, my friend. You can handle anything.

Take some time to journal now

- *Which areas in your life do you need to take a closer look at?*

- *How will you plan to do that with more love, kindness and compassion?*

Chapter 4

Where Are You Now?

My reason for studying nutrition and dietetics in college, even though I didn't know it at the time, was based on a genuine desire to help people design their lives with intention and curiosity as it relates to their unique wellness journey. It wasn't just about the food, and I had no interest in 'fixing' people because here's the truth: You are not broken, and there is nothing wrong with you, ever! Sure, things can be improved, and you can make a change when something feels out of balance, but you are still a whole human being, just as you are. Health is a special journey for everyone, and I wanted to be a part of that! People are fascinating to me, and by listening to and working with others, I continue to learn about myself.

At the time, I had no idea how fulfilling this path

could actually be. I never realized the potential I had to guide people towards change, real change, and results which are more profound than what you get just by telling someone to drink more water and eat more vegetables. As a sophomore in college, when I chose my major, I had no idea that years later I'd be stepping into a role that would allow me to help people create their lives with more confidence, freedom and self-love. My education didn't teach me how to do that. I stepped into that power on account of my own personal experience and desire.

I found a personal passion for learning to improve my health and appearance through food and fitness. But over the years, my definition of health had expanded way beyond what it meant to me when I was 19 years old. Around that time, I was obsessed with eating "right" and overly concerned with how my body looked. That wasn't healthy. I was stressed out, worried about boosting my grade point average, and so scared of not being successful in my career. That also wasn't healthy. I danced 10 hours a week, forced myself to eat less than 1600 calories a day, and then worked out more to compensate for, what I believed meant, overeating. Again, not healthy, and what a waste of energy.

I was doing more and striving for more, but most of my choices were made from fear and a lack of self-acceptance rather than a desire to make a real difference in the world.

My thoughts and actions did not come from a place of unconditional love for myself like they do today. Now I intuitively know how to eat, move, dress, work, learn, rest, play, talk and act like I love myself because I DO.

The road I traveled to get there is how I am able to guide my clients towards living their lives with love, not fear, driving their choices.

After years of studying the physical chemistry, biology, pathology, and nutrition of food… I was so done with numbers and calculations. I wanted more. I needed meaning. There's a lot we don't know and understand when it comes to the human body, and that's okay. There's also a lot that we can't necessarily see, but we know it exists. There was so much that I was not taught in school, but that I knew in my gut was essential to explore if I truly wanted to be of service. I decided to learn more about the emotional and spiritual connections that people experience with food. Based on my own struggle of striving for perfect eating, perfect health, the perfect body, and later realizing how much of my life was consumed by this.

I discovered that health is composed of so much more than what we eat. Healthy, nutritious food is definitely important, but it's not everything.

When a person seeks to find harmony in their life, by considering their physical, mental, emotional, spiritual, social, financial, occupational, and environmental well-being… the opportunities for a person to claim true health and success are limitless! You might think of this as a *holistic* approach as it considers a person's entire being and life experience. Anyone who tells you their approach is "holistic" yet still encourages a strict or restrictive lifestyle plan that is not inherently necessary, or without asking you one hundred questions first… they are missing the point.

Wellness is deeper and more fascinating than what we see on the surface, and just because your physical and mental health are not perfectly up to par does not make you unhealthy. You can still choose to be happy today and live a beautiful life even if you're not perfect. When you focus on what you lack, that is what you'll get. When you focus on all that you already are and all that lies ahead of you, that is what you'll see! And at the same time, if you want to move forward on your journey with intention and have real success, it's important to acknowledge where you are right now.

To help my clients move forward in life, beyond their food and body challenges, I take the time to explore where they are right now, how they got there, and where they want to be instead. Why? Because if you're unhappy with where you are, the only way to change that is to take a different path than the one that got you there.

Using weight loss as an example, most people choose the path of 'going on a diet'. Take a moment to reflect on this: *if diets worked, you wouldn't need to keep coming back to them.*

Many people believe that "different" just means finding a new diet or meal plan to try. A done-for-you food and exercise plan doesn't always consider YOU. It rarely cares for all the essential components that make you who you are and neglecting this can hinder your success or ability to "stick with it" in the long run.

A truly holistic approach touches on your values, preferences, budget, time constraints, stressors, family connections, the stories you tell yourself, how you want to live your life, and so much more. More importantly, diets don't consider your past and current relationship with food and your body. A diet doesn't teach you how to check in with yourself and listen to your body for feedback. Some programs are even designed to train you out of listening to your natural appetite and cravings, and instead, teach you to control them. This is not a good thing, my friend.

Diet culture says, "Do this, not that, and it will work, no further questions. Oh, and if you're not having success as expected from the plan, you didn't try hard enough." *Ouch.*

If a strategy for eating and exercising feels restrictive to you, stressful, time-consuming, mind consuming, or your body responds negatively to the point that you can't keep up with it anymore… It's short-term, unsustainable, and it's not the right way for you. That doesn't mean you failed, and you are certainly not "unfixable." I've heard many women share with me that they feel frustrated after years and years of not being able to "figure out their problem with food."

What if there was no problem?

What if there was truly nothing to fix?

Remember, all results are feedback and simply information to work with. Oftentimes to find what works, you must acknowledge what does NOT work. So, do yourself a favor, LEARN from your experiences. It doesn't matter if you once lost 30 pounds and were in the best shape of your life because you worked out like crazy and you ate strictly clean food for three months… 10 years ago.

What if your life right now doesn't allow for that? Then what? *No, you're not doomed.* There is always another way, and probably a more realistic one.

I believe we all go through seasons of life, some more than others, and I have been exploring this within myself lately. Our seasons shift in ways and at times we least expect. So how can you begin to tap into the wisdom of your body and allow for these natural shifts?

Start with being curious.

Based on what you've done in the past, ask yourself…

What was working?

What really wasn't working?

What can I realistically do today?

Can I allow myself to go slow and take this step by step to turn these new practices into lifelong habits?

Am I willing to stay honest with myself and let go of comparison or unfair expectations?

How would it feel for me to let go of the outcome and simply focus on being present with myself?

These types of questions are where I start when working with a new private client. I guide them with curiosity so they can learn to always stay curious with themselves and, day by day, moment by moment, toss what doesn't work for them now in order to discover what does.

But here's the thing…

You don't know what you don't know.

If all you've ever been told is that eating less and exercising more is the magical path to having the body you want, then you're sadly being fed outdated nutrition information and rules. If you're trying to decide between all the "choices" out there… intermittent fasting, juicing, detoxing, raw food, vegan, keto, paleo, no salt, no sugar, no alcohol, no processed anything, no fucking joy… Then, of course, you're going to feel overwhelmed and confused. If you believe you won't be successful unless you're following a plan, then you will continue to feel helpless and disappointed when someone else's cookie-cutter program doesn't work. If you're constantly looking outside yourself for answers, then take a moment to consider why you feel that's the only way to have success. Is it because you don't trust yourself? *Take a moment to pause and reflect on that question…*

Do you trust yourself?

Take some time to journal now

- *Name all the reasons why you should and can trust the wisdom of your own body.*
- *What has your body done for you? How has it helped you or supported you in the past?*
- *What does your body want you to know? What is it teaching you?*
- *Name the experiences in your past where trusting your gut or following your instincts did lead you in the right direction.*

Taking advice from others has a time and a place. It can be useful. And when nothing seems to be working for you, don't get frustrated with yourself because you are not to blame. It's time to get in touch with your inner wellness guide, the one you were born with. I promise it's there; most likely, you just forgot how to listen to it. Hey, be easy on yourself. We're not given any real manual for life, are we? But you're still here. You're still alive. You are on a beautiful journey, and if you made it this far, it's because you were willing to embrace the hard times, acknowledge the good, learn as you go, and keep going.

It's no different with food and exercise. You're a smart cookie, and you probably wouldn't be friends with someone if they constantly shoved their opinions in your face about how you should live your life… right? Well, then don't let other people tell you how you should eat or move. Not even me, if something I say doesn't resonate with you, put it to the side!

There's more to life than following fake promises in bold font on magazine covers in grocery stores.

There's more to having a body you love than making it burn calories and look fit.

There's more to enjoying food than "getting it right" by trying desperately to eat what's good and feeling bad when you don't.

You get to design your life and decide what healthy and happy looks like for YOU, and you don't have to go on that journey alone. When someone approaches me because they're frustrated with food, lacking energy, stressed out, or unhappy in their body, I use FOOD as the doorway. What lies behind that door is always a mystery for both the client and me, which is why I seriously love what I do and find it so fascinating.

My clients have success with me, not because of what they lose, but what they gain.

My clients have success with me, not because of what they are able to stop eating, but what they are able to find joy in eating.

My clients have success with me, not by doing what they thought they could never do, but by doing what they never imagined was possible.

Unlike the multi-million-dollar companies making money off your need to keep buying from them, I don't subliminally promise that having a different body will solve all your life's woes. Think about it, if they really had the solution, you wouldn't need to keep feeding their piggy bank. I DO promise that living a healthy lifestyle without food rules, restrictions, or making yourself miserable is possible! I promise that my approach is personal. I've never worked with two clients in the same way because no two people are the same.

I also don't promise that you'll be exactly where you want to be in any particular length of time – that is unethical, unrealistic, and unfair, in my opinion, to make those sorts of claims. I DO promise that I show up with everything I have and guide my clients on a positive, effective, meaningful path towards positive well-being, self-love, freedom, and a happier relationship with food. There are no cutting corners in real life, some things just take time, and that's okay.

I believe that diets – unrealistic, over-specific, and impersonal ways of eating – are fear-based, quick-fix strategies. Have you ever heard of the acronym for F.E.A.R. as False Evidence Appearing Real? Losing weight on a short-term diet is just that, false evidence appearing real. We think it works because we see results, but it doesn't *really work.* More than 95 percent of people who follow a diet plan for weight loss eventually gain their weight back and sometimes even more. It's not a true strategy for lifelong success if it isn't sustainable. The only diet that works is the one you can stick to, but some health experts and diet companies will not admit that. We just continue to get the conflicting messages that either we need to try harder, or that a program is simple and easy to follow (even when it's not).

The problem wasn't that you stopped trying or failed to keep up with your strategy…

Have you ever considered that the process for reaching your success in the past was not realistic for you to maintain, flexible enough, or faithfully personalized to YOU? Perhaps losing the weight wasn't that hard, but the real challenge was doing what you needed to do to keep the weight off, and eventually became a source for so much misery and frustration.

I've been there.

I reached my 100-pound goal weight when I was 18 years old, and almost immediately after, I was struck by an extreme fear of gaining back even a pound. At first, I thought my success was too good to be true! Shortly after that, the binge eating started. What I didn't realize then was that my binge eating was a result of restricting food to lose weight. The next several years were torture for me as I watched the pounds creep back on. Eventually, though, I reached a place of loving my body, regardless of the number on the scale. And looking back, if I had resisted everything my body was telling me and continued to do what was necessary to maintain that weight… I would be seriously unhealthy. I would be fatigued, cold all the time, malnourished, hungry, unhappy in my body, anxious, obsessed with food, constantly fantasizing about what I couldn't eat, and who knows what else. I'm so glad I chose a different path. If you can relate to that uncertainty and fear around choosing a healthy and happy body versus choosing a smaller body, keep reading…

Your body is supposed to change and fluctuate throughout your lifespan. It just is. There's no denying or getting around that fact. Change is the beauty and nature of being human, and to experience the natural transformations that we as humans go through is something we can hopefully learn to love and accept rather than despise and punish. Despite what anyone tells you, no one has a perfect solution for this, not even me. But we all deserve to have genuine and honest support with our health and wellness goals.

In my humble opinion, a great coach is someone who is willing to take the time, as long as it takes, to walk their clients' journey with them. A great coach can acknowledge all their clients' successes, especially the small ones, whether they lose weight or not. Everyone knows there's more to health than melting body fat and inches.

Take some time to journal now…

- *What does having a healthy and happy life mean to you?*
- *How can you create more health and happiness in your life today?*

Chapter 5

Self-Awareness

Self-improvement is not about escaping who you are now, it's about expanding upon who you already are. In doing so, you must know where you currently stand. You must be willing to take a closer look at yourself to know what you need and where to go from here. Be kind to yourself, respect your journey, and love yourself unconditionally, even when it's hard. From there, work on developing your awareness and practice self-study.

Self-awareness is nothing more than the study of self. Again, it's about knowing where you are in order to know where you ought to go. Awareness through self-study is the foundation of everything because it gives us the power of clarity. When you look within and practice self-awareness, you gain the wisdom to discover what you need; What you need is not always the same as what you want or feel the pressure to be, do or have. Self-awareness, like mindfulness, is not about changing or fixing anything right away. In hindsight, perhaps there is nothing to fix at all! A mindfulness practice is having the discipline to not get carried away in your discoveries, but to just be with them for a moment and be present with yourself.

Get grounded. Get cozy. Being present may feel uncomfortable at times. Let it be.

If self-awareness is a hot fudge sundae, then the cherry on top is learning how to have awareness without judgment (towards yourself and others) or attachment (as a truth) to any particular thought. Like all things, it takes practice.

What I've realized time and time again as I notice my own thoughts and patterns, is that once you become aware of something, you'll start to notice it EVERYWHERE. You begin to realize how often certain thoughts are actually passing through your mind, and it might, honestly, drive you a little nuts at first. Take a deep breath. You'll eventually get over the hump, and it will become easier to work through the thoughts, reframe them, or learn to let them go entirely as you gain more clarity around how or why they show up in the first place. I've seen from my own experience that the most challenging cluster of thoughts to manage are the ones in which I have absolutely no idea where they originate or what triggered them – like a panic attack at 2am - *why is this happening??* One minute you're sleeping, and the next minute you are wide awake, and the thoughts keep spiraling. That can be frustrating for sure. So, start with what you can. When you're honest with yourself, and you truly pay attention, you'll discover what the sources or triggers of your unwanted thoughts might be. It could be the words or ideas shared from a parent, your friends, your coworkers, the news, the internet, advertisements, social media, magazine models, clothing stores, dating sites… the list goes on. You may not always be able to change your circumstances right away or have the means to run away from your triggers. But you can choose to limit your exposure to them and choose your encounters with them wisely. Most importantly, you get to choose how you let them affect you.

I'd love to share a funny and very real story about the relationship I once had with a food tracker.

At some point during my junior year of high school, I downloaded an app on my phone called MyFitnessPal. By the time I was a freshman in college, I had developed such a close, dare I say *toxic*, relationship with this "resource". We'll call her MFP. I later realized she was one of the major triggers for my disordered eating as well as the fear and obsession I began to have towards food and my body.

When we first met, she innocently declared that she could help me track my food intake and calories because she knew I was interested in eating healthier and wanted to make better food choices. I grew to like her and rely on her so much that it became an addiction! We spent every day together. I never skipped a chance to check in. We touched base every time I decided to put something in my mouth, and it didn't matter what or how much I ate, I had to be honest with MFP. I told her everything. Even on the nights that I found myself binge eating on the couch at 11 pm when my parents were asleep, MFP knew about it. I'll never forget the time I was home during summer break after my first year of college. I would stay up late watching TV most nights, feeling so proud of myself for sticking to my calorie goals and being "good" with food during the day. Sometimes I'd check in with MFP and ask, "Hey, I know I already ate 1200 calories today, but what's another 200? Just a rice cake with peanut butter, it's not that bad, right?" And she'd look at me and say, "No, girl, don't do it! You know... If you eat like that every day for the next three weeks, then you will gain two pounds... Within six weeks you'll gain four pounds. Is it worth it? Don't forget about your goal! You already made it to 100 pounds, don't you dare gain it back!!"

But the urge to binge was so strong, even MFP couldn't stop me. For two years leading up to the shift where I started uncontrollably snacking at night, I was fanatically tracking my calories and trying to eat as little as possible to lose weight - weight that I really didn't need to lose. During that time, MFP and I became so inseparable that every time my parents asked, "Who are you texting? You're always on your phone! We're eating dinner now, who could you possibly be talking to?" They didn't know I was talking to MFP, telling her exactly what I was eating so she could help me to stay on track. And if she didn't have the specific calorie count for my meal, I would take the time to break it down and journal every ingredient in the approximate amounts. Calorie counting became a skill I got ridiculously good at… and it's not something I'm necessarily proud of.

There were some days when I would actually look forward to a binge at night, so I would plan for it by adjusting the rest of my meals that day. I already knew it was going to happen, and sometimes, as much as I hated it, I think I even liked it! Talk about a toxic relationship. I was addicted to the uncertainty, the drama, the fact that I could do it without anyone else knowing I was "breaking the rules". It was a moment in the day I finally got to relax, be wild, out of control, and not perfect. To be honest, my body probably needed the 'extra' calories. But the next morning… Oh man… the shame, the guilt, and the frustration I had towards myself would hit me hard. If someone even mentioned food to me, I would become irritated and react with anger. No one knew I was restricting during the day, everyone just assumed I was 'eating healthy'. But on the inside, I was being so particular about what I ate because I was binge eating at night and I didn't know why.

Now I understand how impossible the binge-restrict cycle was to break. I was compulsively eating at night because my body was deprived, and I'm not just talking about calories and nutrients. I was also depriving myself of nourishment, pleasure, and satisfaction from food. These are biological necessities, and sadly, in today's common healthcare practices they're often overlooked. If you're caught eating something just for pleasure and not nutrition, it's labeled as being "bad" or "having a cheat day" or "indulging". Over time I started choosing to look at food purely as fuel for my body - it was for necessity over desire - and I tried to get away with as little fuel as possible so I could be all the things that I *thought* a smaller body would make me: happy, attractive, beautiful, worthy of a lover's attention, successful, confident, having eternal health.

I got sucked into these false beliefs, like millions of people do, and after years of disappointment I finally chose to believe the truth: Weight loss by itself doesn't do much good for our health and well-being.

It's certainly not the only measure of health, yet most healthcare providers are trained to focus so highly on it. I learned the hard way that having a perfect body and perfect health isn't all we are put on this Earth to achieve! My hope is that you will hear my story and learn to choose a different path towards health, happiness and freedom - one that doesn't involve things or people or thoughts that inspire a toxic or conditional relationship with food and your body.

After several years of battling this binge-restrict cycle, I decided I was DONE letting food have any power over me, which was by far one of the most empowering choices I've ever made in my life.

With self-awareness, I realized that MFP was the primary source of it all. She blocked every possibility for me to have healthy thoughts, feelings and behaviors around food. So, I had to cut her off. But letting go wasn't easy…

The problem with hurtful habits and relationships is that they can be very hard to break, especially if we're unaware of the damage they're causing. Remember how I said my relationship with MFP was toxic? No doubt, it was… She was a manipulative, controlling, judgmental, bitch! If you're reading this and you're the founder of MyFitnessPal, I'm sorry. It's nothing against you, personally… but this app needs to go. Programs and resources like these have been unconsciously underfeeding people and providing false information through black and white nutrition guidelines. It's time we move on to better, more realistic ways of eating and living. Tracking calories for weight loss is old news, it doesn't work sustainably, and it never has. We're humans, not machines! There are as many right ways to eat and right paths to take as there are people in the world.

So, I broke up with MFP. Well… Honestly, I broke it off and we got back together several times. Letting go of what no longer serves you after relying on it for so long is never easy. But once you choose to move on and never look back, you will be so glad you did. Once I removed this thing from my life that contributed so much to the negative thought patterns I was having towards food and my weight, I realized the problem wouldn't simply disappear immediately. Just as behaviors become habits, thoughts become habits too. The app wasn't the only source of my disordered eating, and there's no way we can consciously identify them all! We receive countless messages about food and our bodies that plant themselves in our subconscious minds - messages from family, friends, the media, and the world. I never realized how they were affecting me throughout my young life, but looking back, I have memories of comparing my body to other girls' bodies from as young as four years old. It's not uncommon these days for kids to speak poorly of their bodies and to want to lose weight. It really makes me sad. By becoming more aware of these challenges we face and turning inwards to explore how our choices reflect those ideas from the world, we take back our power.

Self-awareness is so valuable but being conscious alone doesn't make it all go away. Once I decided I wanted a healthier relationship with food and to find a more nourishing lifestyle balance, I also realized there was much more work and healing to be done. But I took the challenge, wholeheartedly! I started to become aware of every thought or judgment I was having around food. The ideas came into my mind surprisingly more often than I first expected. *Why the hell have I been living like this??* I remember thinking to myself.

Whenever I wanted to eat something I once labeled "bad", the old voices started to creep back in… *You don't need that. Too much fat. Too many calories. You worked out today, don't ruin it.* In those moments when all I craved was freedom from the noise inside my head, when all I wanted was to be fully present with my friends, when all I needed was to finally experience just eating without worrying about it for once… I would pause, take a deep breath, and remind myself that **these things in my head are just thoughts**!

Even after all those years, the subconscious programming was absolutely possible to undo. While I was practicing self-awareness to recognize the rules I created for myself and work on letting them go, I also needed to practice patience and kindness towards myself. I had faith in the process.

Remember, finding the source or the trigger of your unwanted thoughts is often necessary so that you can remove it. So, what happens when you do that, and the thoughts keep coming back? While they are just thoughts and they don't define you, they can also be present to guide you towards the things that need more attention. With patience, without judgement and without attachment… Can you learn to listen to your thoughts? Can you allow yourself to get a little curious about where they might come from? These answers might not be so obvious. They might not be right in your face, rather subtle, always there so that you barely notice them. Sometimes the unwanted thoughts and feelings that keep coming back are deeply rooted truths that wish to rise to the surface - deeper parts of your soul that long to be heard and addressed.

Is it Guilt? Where do your feelings of guilt come from?

Is it Shame? What are you ashamed about?

Is it a lack of Self-Love? Why should there be any reason not to love who you are?

These are the types of questions we get to ask of ourselves.

We may not always like what we find, but they are absolutely necessary to explore if we wish to move forward with confidence and peace of mind.

Take some time to journal now

What is keeping you from having the relationship with food, with your body, or with yourself that you desire?

Maybe it's MFP! It could be a person, a thing, a thought or an emotion (like fear or doubt). Dive deep and let yourself explore the different areas of your life where you're feeling stuck, where you need to let go.

Letting go isn't only about releasing what no longer serves you... Letting go of the good can be hard too. But in life, we know we can't hold onto everything forever. People, things, experiences come and go. It's a natural flow that often feels right, and other times, it can feel hard to move on, even when it's necessary.

I bought myself some flowers recently, nothing fancy, just a simple bouquet of red and pink from the store closest to me. This isn't something I usually do; however, it was during a time when I needed them most. It was in the middle of winter after almost a year of physical distancing in our homes because of the pandemic. Believe it or not, I only schlepped myself to the store that afternoon because it was right after Valentine's Day. My first thought was, *"Oh, I wonder if flowers and chocolates are on sale!"* And it gave me a reason to do something random and kind for myself. But I quickly grew an attachment to these flowers, they helped me in ways I didn't expect, and I began to enjoy their company.

My store-bought flowers sat pretty in a vase on my living room table for two whole weeks! I was pretty impressed with myself for taking care of them so well. I'm grateful for each day they gave me color and joy when I walked into the room. But once I could tell they were on their last few days… I went to change the water one last time. When I lifted the vase, about 10 petals fell off. When I took another step, a few more dropped again. I said, *"Okay, flowers, you're ready. Even though I don't want to let you go, it's time, and holding onto you would be selfish. Thank you for giving me two full weeks of your beauty."* And I laid them to rest outside.

When we let go of the old, we make room for the

new. *What are you holding onto that needs to be released?*

Chapter 6

You Are Not Your Thoughts

You are not your thoughts… YOU are NOT your THOUGHTS.

Without trying to get too dramatic… I must have been possessed the night I had my emotional breakdown. The experience literally felt as if my thoughts were taking over my entire being. I couldn't stop them. However, there was a thought in particular that spoke to me so clearly… This idea nearly yanked me out of my misery in a split second. It was like a whisper to myself, from myself, gently reminding me, "You are not your thoughts." In an instant, the beast, the overwhelm, the darkness was lifted out of me. I literally watched it go. Poof… This dramatic shift was so profound to me that "being possessed by my thoughts" is the best way I can describe what was happening to me. When I realized my thoughts were not me, I genuinely felt my entire energy lighten up as if that single affirmation flipped a switch, and I was myself again.

Quieting your mind isn't about resisting the urge to think at all. That's simply resistance, and what you resist will persist. Depending on your thoughts, it can be quite a difficult process to hush all that noise. But once you learn to release the thoughts that aren't working for you and realize your thoughts don't have any power over you unless you let them, you can live your life more at ease as you learn how to manage those thoughts better. Freeing yourself from overthinking and overwhelm, like almost any other practice, is a constant, ongoing, daily practice. Why? Because there will always be more life experiences which will lead to more thoughts. Look at it this way, if you aren't thinking, you're brain dead. I have personally chosen to honor my thoughts with gratitude as an affirmation because they remind me that I am still living. We are human, we're alive, and that's freaking awesome! So, whether you like them or not, they are there, but you are not your thoughts. Remember that. YOU – the you that is your soul, your energy, your being - are the *observer* of your thoughts.

Let me say that again… YOU are not your thoughts. You are the observer of your thoughts.

Oftentimes, we believe that by thinking thoroughly through every detail, every doubt, every possibility, and every "what if," that we can perfect each situation and control every aspect of our lives that way. In fact, it's the opposite. When we over think, over plan, and seek perfection out of Life, we will at some point feel a loss of control when things don't go "our way". Once you realize that you don't have to be in control of everything all the time, that it's okay to be in the unknown (and you WILL be okay), the overwhelm of uncertainty will fade and eventually, you won't be as bothered by it.

I'll never forget the first hot yoga class I ever took.

It.

Was.

So.

Slow...

Seriously. That one hour was the longest, most uncomfortable hour of my day. I wanted to enjoy it; I really did! I mean, every other student there seemed to like it so much, and I swear some were probably addicted! Before this class, I only focused on the yoga sculpt classes that my studio offered, which were high energy, high intensity, loud music-driven, and fun. Although it took me a while to understand the sequence and learn how to use the weights with proper form, I was way more in my comfort zone here than in the hot yoga class. It's hard to notice when your mind is wandering with awesome music holding your attention and a screaming boot camp style yoga teacher encouraging you all the way through.

In this class, the lights were dim, yoga mats were practically on top of each other, the mirrors were fogged up halfway through the class, and the teacher had a way of wandering around the room that looked so graceful, grounded, and assertive. I was intimidated. It felt like I was in grade school again. Growing up, there were several times when a teacher would excitedly ask me to sit in the back of a more advanced level class for an hour one day, halfway through the school year, just to test how quickly I would catch on and then decide if they wanted to move me into that higher level. It was flattering, but terrifying! My school had good intentions, but all the students in that class knew exactly what the teacher was talking about, and all I heard sometimes was a foreign language, feeling hot and red in the face, uncomfortable, embarrassed, and dumb. That's how I felt in the middle of this dimly lit yoga studio, surrounded by 30 other students. They looked so in the zone as the teacher's Sanskrit would roll off her tongue…

Inhale Tadasana, Exhale Anuvittasana, Inhale Ardha Uttanasana, Exhale Dandasana...

What the heck did she say? Ardha who? I panicked and gazed around the room to observe what the students around me were doing, trying not to make it too obvious that I was more lost than a second-grade kid looking for the correct giant yellow bus to get on after their first day back at school. Everyone else knew what was going on. Some of the students were even moving on to the next pose in the sequence before the teacher said it!

I remember watching my thoughts spiral faster as the room seemed to move slower and feel hotter.

Am I doing this right? How is this a beginner class? Man, it's so HOT in here! I can't breathe with all the humidity in this air. Maybe I need more water. Oh, but I shouldn't drink too much yet, or I'll have to pee halfway through class. Crap, are we even halfway through yet? It's SO hot, and I hate sweating. I don't know how much longer I can do this. What if I just walked out now? Would the teacher notice? Is that even allowed? Screw it. I'll just stay and get through it. I'm never doing this again. Why do people love this so much??

At that point in my yoga journey, I was aware that this kind of uncomfortable feeling most likely meant

I needed to keep going because the class was challenging me to grow.

Several years later, I was trained and certified to teach that exact yoga sequence! I realized that we were never holding a single posture for longer than thirty seconds, sixty seconds at most. In fact, there is plenty of movement and flow in this particular class. There are only a few moments of true stillness in the whole hour that last longer than a minute, but when your mind is everywhere else, but the present moment and your body is forced to be still… one, quiet moment can feel like the longest uncomfortable silence of your whole day. When your thoughts are running a hundred miles a minute, that minute can feel unbearable.

My hot yoga experience is a great example of being in a situation where my perceived "threats," including my fear of the unknown, fear of failure, and fear of being judged, pulled me out of living in the present and had me stuck in overthinking and overwhelm. Being in my body was uncomfortable, so I flew to my head… but that can be a scary place too! So, what are we supposed to do when we realize we're having a ridiculous number of thoughts at any given moment? Or rather, how do we make sure we don't give our power away to those thoughts? It starts with the simplest, yet most often overlooked step that we must take:

Self-awareness.

The truth is you don't have to believe every thought you ever have. But it can certainly be beneficial to acknowledge them, witness them, and listen to them. Noticing our thoughts is not the same as believing our thoughts are right, but that they are here for a reason. They can teach us what we believe in our core and guide us towards the challenges that need our attention most. Our thoughts, especially those that feel the loudest, most confusing, random, or intrusive, can help us recognize where we might need to let go of trying to be perfect or in control. The keyword here is to FEEL. You'll know when a thought or a pattern of thoughts is not serving you when it does not feel right in your body. You might start to get hot, dizzy, spacey, or feel a pit in your stomach. You might feel like you want to cry, hide, or run away from something. You might feel an intense anger or bubbling urge to shut off the thoughts, and perhaps you don't know how. That's okay. Be still. Listen.

Whatever that uncomfortable feeling is for you, it's your body's way of telling you to pay attention - to give yourself attention.

Your brain's most important job is to keep you alive. So, what often happens when you are in a situation that feels new or uncomfortable, the brain might interpret your experience as a potential danger or threat. Whether the threatening danger is physically real (imagine your car dies on the tracks and you see a train coming full speed ahead… scary, right??) or the danger is a perceived or imaginary threat (picture standing in front of a room full of strangers giving an important presentation and your boss is keeping a close eye because you're under review… also scary) your brain doesn't know the difference between what's real and what's imaginary. Whenever you sense a fear, a threat, a danger, or an enemy, the response in your body is identical.

When the stress response is turned on, hormones like cortisol and adrenaline flood your body to power up your muscles and your brain in order to get you out of a potentially life-threatening situation quickly. You might experience a racing heartbeat and racing thoughts. You might get super strength and make lightning-fast decisions. This is all fine and good in the short-term, about 5 minutes at most. But when something or someone or a thought is constantly triggering the stress response, even at a low or a moderate rate, this is incredibly damaging to our health in the long-term. You probably won't even realize it's happening. Stress disguises itself in the body and eventually shows up as dis-ease, illness, unwanted symptoms, a challenge with food or your body. Some examples of this are the inability to lose weight or keep it off, an unexplained change in weight or appetite, poor digestion, bloating, fatigue, trouble sleeping, mood swings, irregular period or losing your period completely, headaches, increased potential for food sensitivities, weak immune system, muscle tension, and so much more.

I'll be sharing more about some of the impact that diet culture, false nutrition beliefs, normalized body shame, social media and comparison have had on our overall well-being. But I want to point out a few major stressors on the body that are often underrated and overlooked, since we're talking about it here. Most likely, you or someone you know can relate to at least one of these.

- Over exercise or under eating and poorly compensating with proper nutrition after exercise, for the intention of weight loss.

- Skipping meals or choosing to go unnecessarily long periods of time without eating. This is not a sustainable solution, and it can lead to major health concerns.

- Strictly reducing or eliminating major food groups, types of foods, or macro-nutrients.

- Irregular eating times or patterns

- Eating too fast or eating in a state of stress

- Toxic food and body beliefs. These are obsessive, controlling, fear-based, and often subconscious ideas a person develops about eating and how the body should look which leads to negative self-talk and can greatly affect physical, mental, emotional and social well-being.

- Living as a "human-*doing*", always doing, and forgetting to live as a "human-*being*", and remembering to slow down occasionally, breathe, and just BE.

Your intention should not be to completely eliminate or avoid stress. It's about learning how to live through life's challenges and continue to grow, evolve, and become the greatest expression of yourself. It doesn't help us if we are afraid of stress and view it as a threat. This would be counterintuitive. Instead, notice where in your life you might be able to reduce the amount of unnecessary stress you might be putting on yourself.

When we live in the past or worry about the future, it's impossible to be present NOW. The goal is not to never have another negative thought ever again... Even the most positive people I know aren't perfect thinkers; no one is. Quieting the mind is not about "not thinking" because that is humanly impossible unless you're brain dead.

The intention of living in the present moment is to:

- Practice self-awareness

- Practice patience with yourself; notice your thoughts without attachment; witness your truth without judgment

- Practice mindfulness; constantly bring yourself back to the present moment

- Practice letting go; seek to understand what triggers your unwanted thoughts and behaviors so you can more easily release what no longer serves you

Chapter 7

Mind-House Meditation

Meditation is a practice of mindfulness with a focus on one thing - whether it's your breath, movement, physical sensations, music, etc. There are so many ways to meditate, it's not just one thing and the practice can look very different from person to person. Meditation, put simply, is focusing for a period of time on one thing. This will naturally help you to let go of your thoughts, giving them little to no attention in the moment. Again, this relates to ALL your thoughts. Positive thoughts can be a wonderful part of one's healing journey! I'm a huge believer in the law of attraction and using positive affirmations to change your thinking patterns. At the same time, meditation is a great way to come back to your true self and feel your way through life, which I believe has more power and benefit than *thinking* your way through life. We as humans (especially "human-doings" - no shame, we've all been there) need to practice thinking less and feeling more. Not only for our benefit, but also to benefit the world and the people around us.

Think of your mind like a house and your reality, your life, is outside of the house. If you're looking through a window from inside your mind-house and you don't like the view, simply walk to another window and you might see something different! We call this changing your perspective. First you need to have the awareness that you have the ability to change your view and walk to a new window. However, if all the windows in your mind house are dirty from years of dust, dead bugs and gunk build up, you might not like what you see outside no matter which window you look through. The mess on your windows represents years of old messages, stories, experiences and beliefs that have accumulated. You can choose to hold onto the grime and allow it to distort your view of the world. Or you can make the effort to clean your windows once in a while, wiping away what doesn't serve you - what dulls your view of the world around you. Yes, it takes some work, but it's your choice. How will you take care of your mind-house?

In this meditation, choose your favorite room in your mind-house. It's clean, tidy, and quiet. Let your eyes soften and allow yourself to simply relax and be present. All distractions aside - all sounds like the television and music are turned off, your phone is put away and on silent, pets or children are taken care of.

Allow yourself to let go and be still.

As you're meditating, you'll need some fresh air, so metaphorically all your doors and windows need to remain open. Even if you try to keep them closed, they will naturally open from time to time, perhaps by the wind, and whatever wanders into your mind-house - people, birds, squirrels and flies - all are welcome. These "things" are your thoughts. Let them enter, but don't give them too much attention. The practice of meditation is to stay grounded, calm and to become aware in your favorite room of your house. If you try to force the visitors out, they might get angry and insist on staying put just to pester you a little longer. By getting frustrated, you give your power to them and ruin your own peace.

The practice of meditation is to acknowledge the thoughts, the visitors, that they are there. But you don't have to get up and offer them a cup of tea or try convincing them to leave. The windows and doors are still open, so these visitors will naturally come and go, they won't stay forever. Some of your house guests might even be imaginary - they're not real! In other words, you don't have to believe every thought you ever have. All thoughts are simply thoughts, and as you meditate, you can either hold onto them, or practice letting them go.

Some ideas to reflect on from this mind-house visual meditation:

- *What if you chose to clean your windows once in a while? The more often you reframe your thoughts and change your perspective, the clearer and more beautiful your view of the world can be.*

- *What if you allowed the doors of your mind to remain open? Breathe in fresh air and welcome the beauty as well as the chaos of life.*

- *What if you decided not to believe every thought you ever had? You don't have to give all your power and attention to the ideas that hold you back. You have the power to find inner peace, calm and stillness in your mind. It will become easier with self-awareness and practice.*

Chapter 8

Health is Peace of Mind

Your peace of mind and your entire ecosystem of health are not separate entities. In other words, health, well-being, and happiness are not mutually exclusive. In many ways they depend on one another. We know that feeling unwell or out of balance can affect our ability or desire to show up fully day to day. But it's also true that choosing a method or a way of "fixing your problem" that makes you feel unhappy or burdened (for example, going on a strict diet or an exhausting exercise plan) has the potential to negatively impact your health in the long run. So yes, work on your health and take care of your body. But also, be mindful about HOW you approach this.

Consider your state of mind every time you decide to implement a new practice or change an old habit.

When you're contemplating how to go about making

a healthy change, you can ask yourself the following.

Take some time to journal now.

Choose something you're working on, and pay attention to your gut feelings, not the voices inside your head, as you answer.

- *How does this FEEL in my body?*
- *How does my body respond to this?*
- *Does this bring joy into my life?*
- *How does this affect my mental, social and emotional well-being now and how might it impact those areas in the future?*
- *Is this something I can sustain, and for how long?*
- *Is this way of eating/ exercising/ living truly necessary for me to be healthy?*
- *What else can I try that feels right for me at this time?*
- *Does this honor my personal values and preferences?*

- *Does this allow for flexibility in my life?*

- *Can I forgive myself for not being perfect?*

My intention as a coach is to meet my clients, wherever they are on their journey, to guide them towards greater health and happiness. I strive to ensure my clients gain confidence in their lifestyle choices, keeping their highest goals and values a priority. I help them design the life they want to live - not just for a few weeks or months - for as long as they desire. So, it's really about the life lessons, the WHY behind the goal or practice, so that they can continue to grow and evolve on their own throughout their life and wellness journey. You know the old proverbial saying,

"Give a man a fish and you feed him for a day. Teach a man to fish and you feed him for a lifetime."

Most done-for-you food and exercise plans that exist today don't work because they don't teach us how to be flexible, go with the flow, listen to our bodies, or honor our genuine cravings and preferences. For the same reason that bodies change, consider that what a person desires or needs to eat will change throughout the lifespan, for all sorts of reasons. I teach my clients the skills they need to adapt to the seasons of their life. I teach them how to trust and rely on their OWN inner nutrition expert (their gut) for guidance and wisdom so they can finally stop searching for all the answers outside of themselves and instead feel inside for what they want, need and desire.

You may not be totally thrilled about where you are at this moment, and I can empathize with that. Even if you feel like crawling out of your skin right now, don't worry; I've been there. If you're ready to finally reach a place of unconditional love, self-acceptance, and peace of mind, then you absolutely must learn how to *celebrate* your body, find joy in food, and become fully present with yourself.

So where should you start? Remember, it all begins by practicing self-awareness and getting curious about yourself. Acknowledge and accept where you are in this moment if you truly want to move forward.

Break it down into the different areas of your life - physical, mental, emotional, financial, occupational, environmental, social, and spiritual health.

When I first meet with a new client, I look at all these things! I ask questions to get to know as much as I can about the person in front of me. As I continue to hold space for and get curious with my clients, over time, we can get to the roots of whatever in their life, big or small, is disrupting their peace, therefore disrupting their health.

I have one client who realized through talking with me that a huge obstacle for her was that her chatty pups were affecting any chance of her eating in peace. She hated when her two dogs would bark and beg on either side of her, causing her to feel agitated and rush through her meals. We discovered this during her third session. Again, sometimes the little things are the big things, and it wasn't so obvious at first. She wanted to lose weight and was struggling with this for years. I found out she doesn't eat very much food throughout the day, often having very little appetite or interest in food unless she's cooking for and eating with her family or friends. We had talked about eating slowly and finding the pleasure in food that she loves - embracing the flavors of her culture and giving herself time to savor, process and digest the experience of eating. But finally, we discovered a major piece to the puzzle… She was literally eating in a state of stress every time she came to the table. By taking one extra step to put her pets in the other room, she was able to enjoy her meals, reclaim her peace of mind and take back her health.

Take some time to journal now

- *Where in your life is your peace being disrupted?*

- *Explore the different areas of your life and consider which things, people, places, experiences, thoughts and emotions might be a barrier to your success.*

- *In what ways might this be impacting your health on a physical level?*

Chapter 9

Trust the Journey

I worked with a young woman who was such a delight, and she taught me so much about this one truth that most coaches won't admit: *No one can predict exactly how long it will take for anyone to reach their goals*. No one. Not the expert, not the student or client. Therefore, once again, it is so important to stop buying into the "lose weight fast" and "detox your body in just a few days" crap that the media throws at us. No one has the authority to know and understand your body better than you and God or the Universe or Life, whatever higher power you believe in and however you name it. You probably, in your gut, know this to be true. When we have a goal or an idea in mind, especially when it comes to our health, we usually cannot predict the exact details or timelines for how our journey will unfold. That is the mystery of it and that's what makes life crazy, complicated, and beautiful. We don't have all the answers for why things happen the way they do, and that is okay.

If there is a challenge you have not yet been able to overcome, I believe it's because there is still a lesson to be learned or a truth to be embraced.

My client, we'll call her Maya, was 21 years old when we met. She was struggling with low mood and low energy for several months. She had a history of weight loss, followed by extreme fear of gaining it back, which led her to become obsessed with healthy eating and exercising to stay fit. I connected with her story right away as I saw the similarities in my own experience. However, working with her was particularly interesting because she had already recognized this was a problem for her and had previously done the work to find freedom and flexibility in her lifestyle choices. She started to make peace with food and her body to enjoy eating again, and ultimately have her life back. She was pretty happy with her body and mentioned even wanting to gain a few pounds to be at her *set point.*

A person's set point weight is a comfortable average weight which to that person feels healthy and easy to maintain. Just before working with me, she noticed herself slipping back into her old ways of thinking around food, which led to guilt, judgment, increased irritability, and decreased self-esteem. On top of that, she was dealing with various doctors to navigate a rare digestive disorder that was flaring up badly, affecting her ability to keep food down almost daily. Before this shift in her health, she was studying abroad in Spain having the time of her life. While she was there, she admitted that she hardly experienced any digestive flare-ups and truly enjoyed the abundance of delicious, authentic cuisine. Unfortunately, her trip was cut short due to the COVID-19 pandemic that started quickly spreading in the first couple of months of 2020. All the students had to leave, and even the colleges were shut down or in-person classes, so she ended up living back at home with her mom, dad, and siblings.

Let's just take a step back for a moment… I think any college kid in their 20s would have had a difficult time with this, regardless of their health status or mindset before being sent home to live with their family again. That is stressful, heartbreaking and can certainly have some effect on a person's physical, mental and emotional well-being. She had adventure, independence, freedom, health, happiness… and it was all ripped away from her in an instant. That is a lot to manage.

Navigating life as a college student at home and creating a new routine with her close-knit family who was always close by was without a doubt challenging at first. Through our sessions together, she realized that her lack of confidence and overwhelming feelings of guilt about what she was eating were often triggered by comparison. At times she was stuck in her head, turning into her own food police for wanting to have dessert or have a snack at odd times, especially compared to her mom and sister. Because of her digestive disorder, certain foods were easier for her to digest and prevented nausea, even if they seemed boring, bland, or unhealthy compared to what was on her family member's plates. When everyone else in the house was working out and doing virtual yoga together, she noticed feeling upset with herself, even if she wasn't in the mood to move. She felt she 'should' be working out with them, regardless of whether her body and mind required sleep or school and study priorities! Essentially, Maya was constantly in self-judgment towards what she was or was not doing.

We've all been there at some point…

Consider the moments throughout your day when choices around food or exercise are made from judgment, guilt or shame rather than pure desire.

Our work began with gaining clarity around Maya's unwanted or negative thoughts, particularly on when they showed up and what they were about. From there, it made sense for me to help her create some positive affirmations and mantras, unique to what she was struggling with at the time. She planned to recite them daily, whenever, and however it made sense for her. Over the next several weeks, she really began to embody these affirmations. She started to regain her confidence and control around what and when she wanted to eat that felt right for her body. She got out of comparison mode and felt like herself again.

The reason this client's story stands out to me comes back to the idea that no one can predict the journey and it really can be so different from person to person. Maya returned to that place of peace, well-being and confidence in less than two months… TWO months! My journey to making peace with food and learning how to eat on my own terms, without rules or restrictions, in a way that inspired total joy and nourishment lasted several years from the moment I recognized I was unhappy. On the other hand, I've met women in their sixties and seventies who *still* struggle with the same old things that probably started in their twenties or thirties. Maybe it wasn't until later in life, or maybe they've battled food and their body since childhood! I would guess that too many women end up taking these unnecessary, inner battles with them all the way throughout their life, overlooked and unresolved.

Regardless of how long you've been battling something, it is never too late to get started or start again and it is never impossible to make a lasting change or heal. Whether it's a challenge around weight, body image, poor digestion, obsession with following the latest diet trends and calling it a "lifestyle", anxiety, binge eating, emotional eating, low self-esteem, or confidence that you or someone you know is dealing with right now… Remember this: No one is allowed to tell you how long it should take to overcome that challenge. Your journey is yours, it has a purpose, and it deserves to be walked with intention, patience, and love.

In my practice, I hold space for working with weight and body image, and I intentionally blend them into the same category. For my clients who want to lose weight, sure, I'll help them with that. But you better believe we will talk about body image as well! Here's what I've learned… You might lose all the weight you set out to lose, and still find a reason to feel unhappy in your body or dissatisfied with your life. My story is a great example. I weighed 100 pounds at my lowest, and even then, I didn't feel good enough. As a coach, I refuse to work with a client on their weight unless we also work on body image. How you look and how you feel about how you look are two different things, and in my experience, how you feel is more important. I often hear from women that if they could just lose the weight, they will finally have everything they want. What I'm always curious to know is why they believe that to be true?

What is it about that specific number or that particular shape that you believe will change your life?

- *What will a different body allow you to be, do or have that you think isn't possible now?*
- *How will you be a changed human once you have that body?*
- *What makes you think you can't create the happiness you desire NOW?*

I ask women to get crystal clear when answering those questions because what I see is a situation where women are subconsciously placing conditions on what they want. They believe they can't or won't have that thing they desire until something else in their exterior world changes first. Honestly, there's no good reason to put your life on hold. It all comes down to fear and doubt driving the car, and you're sitting in the passenger seat, deciding that you are not in control or your own happiness or that you don't deserve what you desire. Here's the thing about happiness too… Humans are not biologically designed to find happiness; we are created for survival and reproduction. So, happiness is something you must create for yourself, no one else and nothing else can give it to you. I'm not saying those things don't matter, but we can't rely on them to heal or nourish our soul.

When my clients and I put the pieces together, we often discover that what they really want is not the result of melting body fat. Losing weight is a *placeholder* for the things they would rather not focus on because that is too hard. In other words, doing the inner work that is often necessary to create what you want in life is tough! No one promised it would be easy! It takes great courage to look deep inside yourself, to recognize and reflect on the messy, ugly, honest parts of yourself. If you think eating healthy is hard, learning to love and accept your body is even harder. It takes a greater level of commitment to consciously weed out the negative, manipulating messages we get from the world that say we can't love ourselves unless X, Y, and Z happen first.

But just because it's hard doesn't mean it can't be done.

If I did it, and other humans have done it, so can you! Reaching the greatest highs are often a result of reaching the lowest lows - the ups and downs of life are inevitable, and they're necessary for growth and change. So you can keep going down the road of never-ending frustration and disappointment with food and your body, or you can choose to be brave and take a new approach, a better, more positive, and effective approach of learning to honor your journey, have faith in taking the road less traveled, and create the life you want NOW.

I do want to point out that sometimes, choosing to take care of yourself first can lead to a greater sense of self-worth and confidence, and I do see this happen. You start eating better, moving your body more, doing things that inspire you and the feelings of self-love begin to rush in. You just start somewhere, and you notice the positive effects, so you keep going and keep going, and there's no turning back. From that perspective, yes, sometimes just the acts of self-care can quickly lead to self-love and greater health; there's no denying that. It's similar to how choosing to focus on your positive thoughts can lead to more positive thoughts, like a domino effect.

But creating a healthy, happy life is not always a simple, straight line. What I see happening way more often is that a person decides to start eating better and doing the things that they believe will impact their health first… And even when taking it slow, if they neglect to work on their thoughts and their attitude towards themselves in combination with the "plan," then the judgment, the not-enough beliefs, the perfectionism, and the fear can start to creep back in. This causes them to "fall off the wagon" or slip into their old ways of living that weren't working for them.

In my experience, choosing to love and accepting yourself FIRST is the most effective way to go. When you love and cherish your body, you can't help but want to nourish it, feel it, be in it, let it play and express itself. When you love yourself, self-care becomes a no-brainer and it's easy... Seriously, I see so many women struggling to figure out what the whole "self-care" thing looks like. They're "just not doing it," or they have a hard time creating a "routine." But here's the problem with that... In today's world, Self-Care as a practice has the potential risk of turning into another plan to follow - like a diet! Oy vey! Just how we've turned the simplicity and complexity of "eating healthy" into a done-for-you program. Experts are blasting the media with "just do this, and you'll be healthy and happy forever," which takes away an essential component of creating a healthy, happy life... and that essential component is YOU.

If you Google self-care, you'll probably find things like "The 5 Best Self-Care Practices for Every Area of Your Life" and "12 Ways to Take Better Care of Yourself". In my opinion, it's sad that we even need this type of guidance. Remember the days when we didn't have the internet?? If you're younger than me you probably don't. People took their health and their lives into their own hands and figured it out. We all need help sometimes, so trust me, there's no judgment here. I'm a coach who literally guides people in the kindest way possible on how and when to take the next best step forward, and what that step might be. At the same time, I believe that we have become too out of touch with our own bodies.

We are drawn to quick fixes and instant solutions. We are lost in comparison. We are overworked by a society that urges more money and more productivity. And we are dominated by an industry that thrives on our insecurities, to the point that we sometimes can't figure out how to guide ourselves anymore. We have forgotten our biological human instincts to love and care for our own body and mind, day to day, moment to moment.

When I work with clients who acknowledge they're out of touch with "how to do self-care," we explore what's lacking in their world and WHY. Most of the time, it isn't enough to say, "just do it." We explore deeper and consider why things are the way they are in the first place - how they got to that point. If the self-care you need or want is lacking, is it a self-worth issue? Or is it simply a matter of needing to replace old habits with new ones? Oftentimes, it's not that you need to do more; rather, you need to do less. There is so much busy-ness in our lives that we don't make time for the little things we want to do.

Whether it's to meditate, read, take a walk, journal, pray, or have a nice hot soak with a candle and a glass of wine at night.

Self-care can be all of these things, but it's really so much deeper than that.

Self-care is not always pretty. Sometimes taking care of yourself means looking inside to find what needs improvement. Self-care means knowing yourself well enough to set boundaries with yourself and with others. Self-care means making sacrifices for the betterment of your health and wellbeing. Sometimes self-care means putting YOU first. As women, we're often taught to put everyone else before ourselves… Our friends, family, children, career, and the community. As women, we sometimes feel that we come last, and the media certainly doesn't help with this. Self-care can be advertised as self-indulgence, when that really is such a surface-level way of approaching it.

If putting yourself first seems like a big no-no or something you have not done in a while, then look at it this way… *When you know how to take better care of yourself, you can take better care of others*. It's also true that you really can't love someone else to the fullest until you learn to love yourself unconditionally. You put the two together, self-love and self-care, and you've got a woman who knows herself, knows what she wants, and knows exactly how to make it happen. But don't let that scare you. You are more powerful and capable of what you desire than you realize! Make loving and accepting yourself a priority so you can learn how to care for yourself properly. It may take some trial and error, it may take longer than you think, and it may look different than you expect. If you're not sure where to start, I would be more than happy to hold space for you so you can practice getting curious, become more self-aware, learn how to trust your body, trust your journey, and have some positive support in the process.

Take some time to journal now

- *What would happen if you let go of the outcome or timeline for your goals and instead focused on creating more trust within yourself?*

- *What would it mean to you if you could learn to love or respect yourself more through the process of reaching your goals, even before or if you ever "get there"?*

Chapter 10

Practice Patience

While thoughts are just thoughts and they don't define you, it's not necessarily helpful to ignore them either. Thoughts and feelings are often connected, and what you continually push down will eventually find a way to resurface. It is beneficial to pay attention to your recurring thoughts, and for the ones that you feel are unproductive or negative, you can learn how to give them a little TLC, reframe them, or guide them in a completely new direction. Listening to your thoughts holds a lot of power and potential to gain wisdom and knowledge for your life. It can help you to understand what's really going on beneath the surface. Sometimes thoughts are crystal clear, and sometimes thoughts are cloudy. They can show up as unexplainable feelings that leave you completely confused about what's actually happening. Or perhaps a million thoughts are rolling around in your head at the same time, and it sounds like gibberish. All you know is that something doesn't feel right. It might come across as feeling overwhelmed, frustrated, irritable, etc.

Reflecting on my emotional breakdown, again, I was angry and upset and frustrated. I felt incredibly alone and confused and helpless. The thoughts were so loud, but they were muffled - being released from so deep in my subconscious that I didn't fully understand what they were conveying at that moment. I'm no psychologist, but I know that a large portion of our daily thoughts, behaviors, and actions are driven by subconscious programming. Ways of thinking can become so habitual we may forget the thoughts are even there. Uncovering this can take a while, sometimes months or even years of listening to your thoughts, before you get to the root of where they come from so that you can change the pattern. Once you find the undesirable patterns you want to change, you'll probably want to have had them fixed yesterday! Be patient, my friend. Patience and non-judgment are really important skills to develop, if you want to have success with this.

These are two of my favorite practices that I remind myself and my clients often because impatience and judgment show up all the time, and they hold us back. How so? People want to grow, but they don't want to be unhappy. In other words, growth is hard. We know this, and it's why so many people would rather stay comfortable in their habitual ways of thinking, behaving and complaining about it… rather than do the dirty work it takes to make a change. I can be guilty of this too! When we feel like something is taking too long, we get frustrated. When we believe something isn't the way it should be, we get defensive and resist it. But the truth is, we are not the ones who get to decide our timeline or how things are supposed to be. I always say things don't happen to us; *they happen for us*.

Even if you don't believe in a God, the Universe, Spirit, or a Higher Power, you know in your heart that you're not fully in control of your life. None of us are! And we shouldn't try to be, I've learned that the hard way, and I used to have a lot of resistance towards that. There is something greater than us out there, and now I fully believe and trust in it, which is partly why I have such a hard time writing goals, for example. It doesn't feel as productive for me to set goals the way other people say it's supposed to be done - by making them specific, measurable, and time-bound. Instead, I focus more on my intentions, manifesting how I want to feel and what I want to create for myself, for others, and in the world around me.

It was about a year after graduating college when I realized it was time to release my attachment to the details around how and when things happen - when goals are met, when success is accomplished, when a new page is turned - because we truthfully don't have all the answers.

In 2017, I was working on my applications, for the second time, to be accepted into a dietetic internship. This is a highly competitive program with a low acceptance rate in which a student needs to finish if they want to sit for the exam to become a registered dietitian nutritionist. I wasn't even sure I wanted to have the title of Registered Dietitian Nutritionist since the career opportunities I already had with my degree were great. It turned out that I was denied an internship again and I felt devastated. But I also felt somewhere deep in my gut that there had to be a reason for this, and those reasons presented themselves to me over the next several years. If I had persistently kept on the path that wasn't meant to be, I might have gotten there eventually, but I probably would have been unhappy in my career. Because I chose to trust the signs the Universe was sending me and moved forward on a new path, it led to what I do today, and I couldn't be happier!

Suppose you're a goal setter, great! Do what works best for you. But I learned that it doesn't really work for me, at least for this season of my life. I do set goals and trust in the power of declaring what you desire. However, my personal approach to that has changed. In my experience, I've been disappointed by being too attached to the "plan" for reaching my goals. Whereas letting go of specific outcomes and trusting that the Universe has my back has opened my vision for what's possible. Practicing patience and trust has led to so many opportunities, especially in my career and relationships, that I never imagined would happen exactly when or how they did, and they have changed my life for the better. So, remember that healing takes time, and the journey looks different for everyone. Comparison and attachment usually set people up for disappointment, whereas trusting the process and letting go of trying to control everything is so freeing. I promise great things will happen when you lead with your heart.

The fact that you're even reading a book like this is BIG. You are choosing, with intention and bravery, to take the next step in your life. Like a spiral staircase, you may not be able to see the very top, but you know the value in taking one step at a time until you get there.

Patience will be your best friend along the way, and remember, it really is a daily practice. I used to get so frustrated with my dad for calling me impatient when I was a teenager. In his own impatience, he would often say to me, "You're so impatient!!" and that only made me more annoyed. Like most high school girls, I had my moments, heated with attitude and a desire to be right. Looking back, I don't think I ever really understood what the word impatient fully meant. Today, I like to think that I'm much more grounded, centered, calm, and have been acknowledged and appreciated many times by colleagues, clients and friends for being so patient with them. Sure, I still get impatient at times, but no one is perfect.

Notice when you might get impatient with your own thoughts, emotions, or behaviors. It will be helpful to find what brings you back to the present - grounded, centered, and calm. For me, those tools are most often breathing, taking a walk, listening to good music, or simply reminding myself to trust the Universe. I'll often close my eyes, take a deep breath in, exhale, and listen for what I need to hear in that exact moment. I'll create an affirmation around it and repeat it to myself as many times as it takes to believe it and feel at peace again. The power in listening to your thoughts is that the more you pay attention, the quicker you'll be able to recognize when you're floating aimlessly and ground yourself again. When you feel stressed out, reframe your negative thoughts into positive affirmations.

Take some time to journal now

Do you know what impatience feels like in your body? Explore the experience and write about it so you can start to catch your triggers before they spiral into overwhelm and frustration.

- *Do you know what patience and surrender feel like in your body? Write it out.*

- *What usually helps you to get into that grounded state of mind? It could be taking some deep breaths, going for a walk, initiating a break, journaling, calling up a friend or a mentor, taking action or even setting boundaries... Make a list of tools that you can reach for when you start to feel impatient or overwhelm*

Chapter 11

Let Go of Your Perfection Expectation

It's scary, isn't it? Starting something new without knowing what to expect? Without having a clearly written plan or process to envision exactly how it's all going to unfold? So, maybe you're the type of go-getter who creates a "game plan". You think through all the "what ifs" and "how-tos" and decide ahead of time how you're going to handle your worst-case scenario, should it happen, *oh but it won't*, and then it does… You watch all your perfect expectations you had of yourself crumble right before your eyes.

Well, here I am writing my first book. I had this amazing idea to put my story onto paper. I'll simply write down all the words of wisdom I've ever shared with my friends, family, clients, and students. I decided I'll gather up all my best content and put it into one place so that someone can discover their own journey towards self-love and acceptance and create a life they love. I thought, *this book is going to be* ***perfect****! For me, writing is a piece of cake, and I already know what I want to talk about. I'll just let it all flow into a beautifully formatted book, and I'll magically have this done in no time. That sounds reasonable... Right?? Great, let's get on with it!*

And then...

Writer's block.

That dreadful thing I've heard about but never imagined I would actually experience myself. I almost always have something to say. Often too much to say, in fact! Why am I sharing this with you now? Because the exact thing I want to write about is the actual obstacle that's holding me back from writing at this moment: *perfection expectation.*

The fear of not being perfect is a sneaky one. It shows up in ways and in places where we might not always recognize it. The first time someone told me to my face that I was "struggling hard with perfectionism" I was so offended! How dare they say that to me? I'm not perfect and I don't intend to be. However, the reality of not living up to my incredibly high expectations of myself has stopped me in my tracks more than once.

So, after staring at a blank screen for nearly five minutes, unsure where to start, I said to myself, "*Alright Lindsey, this is ridiculous! Let go of how you think this should be written, trust the process here and just write what's in your heart. STOP OVERTHINKING for once in your life and just have fun. START SOMEWHERE.*"

So here we are. That's what I wrote.

I've had several of my clients admit to me that they have a fear of failure.

Fear of failure, or fearing anything really, is stressful to the body and mind. Whenever the brain senses danger, threat, something that could be harmful to us physically, or even mentally and emotionally, the body goes into a stress response in order to "fight off" or get away from that thing. Unlike our ancestors, we no longer need to fear going hungry by not making a kill in the wild or being eaten by a tiger in the process… In society today, we typically have very few physical threats to fear, therefore our subconscious mind tends to make up new things to worry about! When the danger isn't physically real - when it's something in our minds that we perceive as being harmful - it's much harder to escape without having conscious awareness of it and doing the inner work to change the story we're telling ourselves. These are also known as self-chosen stress triggers. The good news is, you have the power to defeat them before they have any effect on your health and well-being.

So, ask yourself…

What if there was nothing to fear?

What if you decided to catch yourself in the act of feeling afraid or worrying about starting something new and uncertain?

Instead, choose to be *excited* and take on that new adventure with enthusiasm! Fear and excitement are two emotions that produce the same chemical response in the body. When your muscles tense and your heart rate goes up, you can decide which emotion you want to take over - fear or excitement. You can choose to let fear control the wheel or allow excitement to overpower that fear, creating an entirely different state of mind and experience.

What I've learned from others, and now completely understand from personal experience, is that overthinking and intense anxiety about doing something wrong most likely comes from one thing… Perfectionism.

I believe that a person's desire for perfection is a spectrum. On one end of the spectrum is someone who does not give a damn about literally anything, often settling for the bare minimum, and on the other end is someone who seeks nothing but excellence from everything and from everyone, especially themselves, to the point where nothing is ever good enough. Maybe, like me, you lie somewhere in the middle. This could mean that you have the awareness that no one and nothing in life is perfect, so there's no sense in trying to BE perfect. However, that doesn't necessarily stop the subconscious desire from influencing our overall well-being. Much of our thoughts, beliefs, doubts, and worries are still rooted in the story that we are not good enough. Perfection can also be described as having a rule or value that if something isn't done *the way it's "supposed" to be*, then it's wrong, bad, or unworthy of acknowledgment. This way of thinking closes us off from seeing another path, another way, another road to success.

Where I see so many of us falling short when it comes to our health and well-being, is believing that the method or action plan must match everyone else's. When in fact, there are as many right ways of eating on the planet as there are people! The "right" way is YOUR way. You will absolutely get it wrong before you see success. So…

What if failure wasn't real?

Thomas Edison said, "I have not failed. I've just found 10,000 ways that won't work."

It's all about perspective and you can choose to believe anything you want. Instead of thinking that nothing you do is ever good enough, or that you fail every time you start something new… Why not instead believe that it's not possible to fail at anything? If you decide to show up as the best, most authentic, most honest version of yourself, then you cannot fail. But of course, it all depends on how you look at failure.

Some people believe the only way you can fail is if you never try. Others use their failures as motivation to work smarter or to inspire growth in a new direction. But the reason I'm discussing it here is based on an observation I've made with my clients over the years who use the words "I failed" way too often. They might even say it unconsciously - and certainly not in a reflective kind of way, rather it comes from a place of deep shame. They look at the mistakes they've made along their wellness journey as a sign of weakness, or that they themselves are a failure.

Words are powerful. The more you use words of judgment like "failed," "should," "wrong," "trying," "can't," etc.... your body listens, it responds, and your subconscious mind holds onto them. Making mistakes and failing at something are not the same thing. We all slip up or make the wrong choice at times, and we can choose to learn from that experience. But I don't consider any part of that process to be a "failure."

Think of this instead... "*It's not a failure; it's feedback.*" I don't know who said this first, but I honor that statement and stand by it. Whether for my personal goals, business goals, or relationship goals, failure doesn't mean we're doing it wrong. Failure aims to guide us in a different direction. The problem occurs only when we become so afraid of what we might discover from that feedback, that it keeps us from getting started in the first place. You might feel worried that you'll mess up so bad and only make things worse. Sure, maybe. But what if you have it in you (and you do) to make things inconceivably better! YOU have the power to decide what is right and what is wrong for you. Right?

So just. Get. Started.

I have memories of being in an art class in my middle school days where fear and perfection often stood boldly in my own way. I loved art. I was good at it, and I've always enjoyed the times where I had the freedom to explore my creative side. Every project was new and exciting, some more challenging than others. But still, my fear of not being perfect was stronger than my excitement. If I were ever unsure of where to begin on a new project, I would just sit there, wide-eyed, hands trembling, staring at my blank canvas in fear. While all the other kids around me were going for it, trying different things, and some were even halfway done with their task for the day… I was so afraid of messing up or doing it wrong that I couldn't even start - as if making a mistake would be the end of it and I'd have to start all over from scratch. But the only person who could ever critique my art as a "failure" was ME.

We are our own worst critics.

I challenge you to get curious about where your perfection comes from. What drives your desire to perform based on overly specific or unrealistic expectations of yourself? This isn't about staying where you are and avoiding growth. Of course, we want to strive for more and become the best version of ourselves, in each and every moment. But you must always remember that who you are now and what you are capable of TODAY is more than enough.

You will absolutely make mistakes along the way. You will need to explore many variations and discover what doesn't work for you in order to find what does. Can you allow yourself to be okay with that?

Nothing in life is perfect, and that is what lies beneath the beauty of it all.

Take some time to journal now

- *Consider a time in your life in which you approached your health or well-being without the pressure of perfect expectation*

- *How did it go?*

- *How did you feel?*

- *What were your wins or successes?*

- *What did you discover by surrendering to the natural flow of your unique journey?*

Chapter 12

What's In Your Closet?

When you feel good, you look good. That's my unpopular opinion. It's much more common to believe that only if and when we *look* good on the outside (according to some arbitrary standards of beauty), then we will feel good about ourselves. While that can be true, it shouldn't be the default pathway for feeling good, even though it probably is for most people. The connection between how we look and how we feel is a two-way street, and if we let it, the less popular direction can become the default. Contrary to what you might have been told, you don't have to wait until you have a 'perfect body' to feel like magic. It is definitely possible to feel great about yourself today!

Don't believe me? Think about happiness. Science proves that smiling can literally change the chemistry in your body in a matter of seconds by releasing neurotransmitters including dopamine and serotonin that help reduce stress and positively impact your mood. In other words, you don't have to wait until something outside of yourself makes you happy for the corners of your mouth to lift. Smile first and observe how your mood changes! Feel good-looking, beautiful, sexy, and confident first, and watch yourself transform before your eyes!

A woman is a queen in her energy and spirit. But only when she chooses to step into her queenhood fully, embracing all of who she is beyond her physical appearance, and she is able to fulfill her greatest, most powerful potential. That woman can walk into any room with a bright smile, bringing their positive energy and their confidence everywhere they go. Not because they're special or any better than you, but because they choose to own who they are and uphold every part of their being.

You can be that woman, no doubt about it! A queen, sitting with pride and assurance on her throne, already lives inside you. You must be willing to let her shine.

Have you ever met someone who has everything going for them on the outside…? A great body, good health, a loving family, a stable job, a successful partner, and they still appear unhappy or unfulfilled like nothing is ever good enough? It goes to show that happiness doesn't come from the things we have; it comes from within. We've all felt that way at some point, right? Hiding behind our to-do lists, our excuses and our Instagram filters, just waiting for the 'right moment' for our truth and presence to be known - waiting until we have that one thing we want so badly, and only *then* can we allow ourselves to be happy and celebrate our lives. But your life is happening today, my friend, and you are already worth celebrating! Don't wait for that day, that moment, or that one thing to arrive (whether it be the better body or the luxurious lifestyle) before you choose to have, and do what makes you feel right and whole, now.

I've seen people procrastinate in their dating life, because they feel they don't yet have the body they need to embrace their confidence and be attractive to the person of their dreams. You are beautiful enough and good enough already, and you deserve to be with that person now! Anyway, wouldn't you rather be in a relationship with a partner who loves you for YOU, and not just your looks? An ideal partner would adore your personality, your heart, your mind, your dreams, and your values. So why are you letting your body determine your worth? Why would you allow anything to stop you from claiming what you already deserve? Go after it, friend! Besides owning your real beauty and talking yourself into believing your worth (because honestly, it's not always that easy) let's talk about what else you can do to feel at home in your own skin.

When a person feels good about themselves, everything around them changes for the better. When you feel good about yourself, your smile shines brighter, you take compliments with grace, clothes feel better on you, and I'll even go so far as to say that food tastes better when you feel good in your own skin!

There are many ways I help my clients around their weight and body image, and I appreciate how each client's journey is so unique.

What's in your closet?

Have you ever walked into your closet or opened your drawers, stood there with your arms crossed, and thought, "I have nothing to wear," as you gaze with disappointment at piles and hangers full of clothing? Your clothes do say a lot about you, and most women underestimate the impact that what's in their closet has on their body image - the visual perception of one's own body.

I've met very few, if any, women who love their bodies so much that they wouldn't change a thing. I am proud and grateful to admit that I am one of them, but it took me years of patience, kindness, forgiveness, and willingness to step into the unknown of my healing journey to get there. I love the skin I'm in, and that has nothing to do with the number on the scale, the inches around my belly, or the size of my jeans! My relationship with my body isn't perfect, and I don't expect yours to be given the world we must face together. I still have my down days, but one thing I can say for sure is that when I'm feeling good about myself and my life, my body image reflects that! So many people have bought into the story that once they have the body of their dreams, *then* they'll be happy. What a load of crap that is! I learned the hard way, so you don't have to. You are more than a body, and at the same time, making peace with your body is a great place to start in order to finally get out of your head about it and actually live your life, embodied.

The most intentional people I know are embodied, meaning they feel at home in their own skin. They live in their body more than they live in their head. If you're not okay with being in your own body, how could you possibly teach others to be? While talking with my yoga mentor, Jill, one day, I asked her why she believes such a small percentage of the students who go through yoga teacher training actually become teachers in the end. Through our conversation we concluded it's because they get locked in their own heads. They overthink the words to stay or lack confidence in carrying themselves across the floor, unable to guide a room in part due to their own fear of not doing it perfectly. To be a great yoga teacher, you don't have to be perfect, because you never will be. To tap into the intuitive nature of guiding someone else's body with love and kindness, you must know how to be present in your own body with love and kindness.

Just before that conversation with Jill, I was stretched out on my yoga mat in Savasana at the end of a great yoga sculpt class that she taught. As I lay still with my eyes closed, I had a moment with myself, appreciating how magical it felt to be completely quiet and totally present with my breath, in my body, at peace - a feeling I didn't always have in my life - a way of being with myself that took years of self-awareness, trust, patience, letting go of perfection and committing to love myself unconditionally.

When you refuse to love yourself, and the less willing you are to connect with your body, as it is right now, the harder it will be to slow down your thoughts. Because if you're not comfortable being in your body, the only other place to be is in your head. Yoga as a practice is all about embracing the mind-body connection.

Vinyasa is a Sanskrit term. It means breath synchronized movement - a meditation, it's about being fully present at the moment, fully conscious of your breath and your body moving as one. When you are fully focused on this, it's almost impossible to hear your thoughts because you can only focus, truly focus, on one thing at a time.

I saw a meme once that showed two words: DIET and HEALTH. Highlighted within these words were the words DIE and HEAL. Whoever created this meme made a sarcastic (but very true) comment: never trust something that has the word DIE in it. Health is about healing, not dieting. I remembered thinking how clever that was. As I typed the word embodied, that same concept came to mind. But this time, what if the word DIE that you see highlighted within the word, embodied, symbolized the death of your thoughts? By choosing to be IN your BODY, you release your thoughts from having any power over you because you no longer choose to focus on those thoughts.

Breathe that in for a moment.

As a coach, I will spend some time getting to the bottom of my clients' strong desire to change their body as I try to understand what they believe will happen once they do. We might talk about what inspired that idea and what they believe is holding them back. I get curious with my clients. I ask them enough questions to get crystal clear around their deeply rooted desires because sometimes, I'm not sure they really know the 'WHY' until we explore it together.

My goal is to guide my clients towards what they really want. Often what they really want is not a perfect body or to be given a flawless diet… and they know this. They want to feel more confident, reassured, full of energy, have more fun, more adventure, more freedom, and be more present so they can enjoy their life and the people in it.

They realize quickly while working with me that achieving those goals usually looks very different from their expectations of health and success. You know my story… I worked so hard to weigh 100 pounds, thinking it would make me more likable, sexy, happy, confident, attractive, and I thought I'd finally be so in love with my body that I'd never have another negative thought about it again. Once I reached my goal weight, I was even more self-conscious of how I looked and lived in fear of gaining the weight back.

When my clients tell me they want to lose weight, I ask them why. This allows them to dig deeper than a surface level problem to realize what they really need in life. I also ask this question for myself, as it provides insight for guiding my client in the right direction so they can achieve all the things they truly want to have, feel and be.

Here's an example:

I want to lose weight... Why?

Because I don't feel confident in my body... Why?

Because every time I try on clothes, I hate how I look... Why?

Because the clothes I buy end up being the wrong size or they just don't fit right... Why?

I don't know, because I really like certain clothes and I just want my body to fit them... Why?

So, I can feel good about my body in the clothes that I wear.

This was an exact conversation I had with one of my clients. Together we are working on her personal challenges around weight and her image of herself. A valuable *Aha* we discovered together in this conversation was that her *clothes*, the lifeless pieces of fabric hanging in her closet, were a huge trigger, affecting her self-worth and happiness. She has a closet full of items that aren't working for her...

some she had bought years ago and kept them around thinking, "maybe one day I'll be able to wear it." It's no wonder she has so many doubts and negative thoughts about her body! She is triggered every morning as she dresses in her own clothes. Her wardrobe currently represents all the "shoulds" and "what ifs" about her body and her lifestyle, rather than supporting her in embracing the queen that she is. How you feel about what you wear matters - it can either make or break your confidence. I reassured her that clothes are not created equal to size - I learned this from a fashion consultant and my client didn't know this… most people don't! Different brands and designers use their own measurements to determine how they want to label a piece of clothing. I'm no wardrobe expert, but I do know that wearing brands and styles of clothing that compliment your body shape will make an incredible difference in how you feel in your clothes. Find the clothes that fit your body, don't buy clothes with the hopes that your body will fit into them.

Imagine a world where clothes in stores didn't have numbers on the tags, and you just had to try on fabric until you found something that fit right and complimented your body well. Realistically, this could easily lead to chaos and frustration without having some sort of guiding system… However, we would for sure experience a lot less comparison and body shame. We wouldn't even have the option to torture ourselves against the numbers, which can either make or break our confidence for the day, the month, the year…

As women, we're swayed by the fashion and diet industries constantly. It's up to us to recognize our worth and not give our power away to a number labeled on a piece of fabric! The next time you're trying on a new outfit, remember that the clothing tags do not determine your value as a human being. And since we're talking about clothes here, consider that who you choose to go shopping with should also reflect how you want to feel about yourself. I'm not suggesting that you start comparing yourself to every friend you have… Just note how you've felt in the past as you try on clothes in a dressing room. Were your thoughts and feelings about your body influenced by who you were with? Who in your world makes you feel like a *Rockstar* when you strut out of the dressing room? If you can't think of a single person, then maybe it's time to shop alone or find some more body-positive friends to hang with. You can count me as one of them!

To help my client literally *feel lighter* in her clothes, we talked about clearing out her wardrobe of anything that doesn't make her feel fabulous. This is a journey, and I know it's going to take time. It's not that easy for everyone to just ditch the clothes they've got, especially if they spent a good amount of money on them. But it makes no sense holding onto things that don't serve you and weigh you down. You can donate the clothes, return the ones that still have tags, exchange them for money or give them away to friends.

Be honest with yourself on whether you need to freshen up your wardrobe. This is all about giving yourself a clean slate, only keeping the clothes you feel amazing in. It really doesn't matter if it's in style according to the fashion industry, and it doesn't matter what other people think about them. It only matters how you feel about your body when you slip on every piece of fabric you own.

Upon further reflection of this spring cleaning and wardrobe clearing process, we discovered something that I want to make very clear here as I did with my client. When you're looking to feel good in the clothes that you own or try on in a dressing room, it will take some serious personal reflection to know the difference between a *clothes* issue and a *body image* issue. Take note of your initial thoughts when you put on clothes so you can reflect on them later.

Take some time to reflect on these questions. Which scenario sounds more like you?

- *How often do you consider that a clothing item simply doesn't compliment or flatter*

- *your unique and beautiful body the way you want it to, so you move on to the next outfit without a second thought about the value of your body?*

- *How often do you stand there, gazing in the mirror, feeling unsure, picking apart your body, and deciding on all the reasons for why you should or shouldn't wear that thing as you proceed to declare all the ways in which your body is wrong because it doesn't fit in THAT clothing item?*

The first is a clothes issue, and that's usually much easier to handle. The second is a body image issue which is built on years and years, sometimes decades, of stories and body shame. We can't expect to undo all that messaging and programming overnight. But it IS possible when you know where to start. Taking a deep and intentional look at your wardrobe, and acknowledging yourself with love and kindness, is a great place to begin.

You don't have to replace everything right away… Can you be okay with just soaking it all in for a minute? Can you allow yourself to know what it's like to be surrounded only by clothes that make you feel like a rockstar? Even if your wardrobe becomes very minimal, it's temporary. Can you just be, and embrace this newfound feeling of lightness?

Moving forward, I challenge you only to buy clothes that you love and fit you at that moment. Not for the body you *want* or *think* you'll have someday… Wishing for "someday" is not being kind to your present self.

If your wardrobe had a voice, I bet the clothes that don't fit are saying something like, "Oops, not yet! Your body still isn't good enough for *me*. You'll have to work a little harder to get into this bad boy."

Ouch! Don't let clothes talk to you that way! Never let anyone talk to you like this. You're better than that. Not all clothes are made for your body, and that is okay. In fact, most clothes are designed and made using mannequins, not real
bodies. Think about that for a moment.

This is your body. Honor it. Take care of it. Embrace it. Own it. Let it shine!

Chapter 13

Let Your Body Shine for You

Time to Play!

Now that we've talked about doing it... Let's take action. Go to your closet and put together an outfit of your favorite clothes. You know, the pieces of fabric in which every time you put them on, you feel beautiful, sexy, comfortable, like you can do anything! I don't care if it's that "little black dress" or your favorite leggings and an old t-shirt. Go ahead and even put on your best shoes, your favorite undies, the accessories that make you feel on fire. Put on YOUR favorite outfit to remind yourself of your power. Dance in it. Strut your stuff in it. Walk down the street, in your kitchen, anywhere you like! Go out to dinner with your favorite person wearing it. Create something spectacular wearing your outfit. Point to yourself in the mirror and say, *I've got this... I AM UNSTOPPABLE!*

Do it all. Feel like the badass that you are. I don't care how cheesy it sounds. You'll feel amazing! Just thinking about doing this for myself right now makes me smile. Try it on and make a note of how you feel afterwards. Again, your goal moving forward should not be to fit into the next size down. It should be to wear the clothes which give you *that* feeling. Wear your new wardrobe proudly with confidence.

I've said it before, and I'll repeat it time and time again… what you focus on grows. So, if what you lack is front and center, that is what you'll see. If you focus on building love and gratitude for yourself, it will flourish and grow stronger each day.

Affirmations are an intentional and powerful way to call in what you need. They can especially guide us towards believing and embodying the things about ourselves that we may not think are true just yet. It all comes down to the stories we tell ourselves. I used to say about myself, for example, that I'm not a good public speaker. I only said that because I would feel so nervous standing up and talking in front of people, even when everyone else thought I did a great job. I was too hard on myself, and I still can be at times. But I refuse to believe anymore that I suck at speaking, so my personal affirmation to embody my truth is, "I am a confident and knowledgeable speaker. People are ready to hear my message and are drawn to my positive energy." I say it every morning before I give a presentation, guide a workshop, meet with a new client, or before I have a difficult conversation. The more I say it, the more I feel it. Words really do have that much power!

Take some time to journal now

What do you like, love, or truly appreciate about your body?

Does anything come to mind right away? If the answer is yes, take a moment to write it down. Post it on your bathroom mirror, make it your iPhone background, recite it out loud as an affirmation before each meal… Do whatever you need to do so that you are reminded of what you love about yourself daily! Write down one, two, maybe three things you can honestly say you love about your body and WHY.

If the question, "What do you love about your body" is uncomfortable or difficult to answer… I want to help you take a closer look at what's beneath the surface so you can finally let go of what isn't serving you and embrace the body you have. The common error I see most clients make when asked this question, that initially holds them back from seeing their real beauty, is that they are only focused on the outward physical appearances of their body. However, your body is much more than what we see on the surface! If you've spent years, or even decades, criticizing yourself in the mirror and comparing it to unrealistic, celebrity bodies on social media… of course, it will seem impossible to even come up with ONE positive thing you can say about this body you inhabit.

Be intentional and get quiet with yourself. Take purposeful time to honor your journey, appreciate where you've been and where you're going; Appreciate your body for all it *does* for you - how it moves you throughout this life and how it works so hard with all its efforts to keep you alive and as healthy as it possibly can; Respect your mind and how it keeps you alive; Acknowledge everything you are capable of doing, having, and being in this body.

I am working with a client now, a woman in her early 20's, who claims to struggle with body dysmorphia; this was the term she used to describe her challenge. She feels frustrated by never feeling sure of what she sees in the mirror, not knowing what is "real" or in her head, and often seeks reassurance from others to confirm if she *looks okay*; deep down exists a powerful urge to constantly prove to herself and others that her body is 'good enough'.

While I do not and have never claimed to be a practitioner who treats body dysmorphia or eating disorders and the like, she is happier to receive my guidance focused on body image while improving her relationships with food and with herself. During one of our recent conversations, I challenged her to the next level of self-awareness when she brought it up. I essentially said, *what if it really didn't matter what you looked like?* Her answer? "I wish." So, I said, "You don't have to wish, you can make this your truth! Believing we need our bodies to validate us is a programmed message that we absolutely have the power to change. It's only true if we decide it's true."

Since she had done quite a bit of work already on exploring her power, her worth, taking ownership of what makes her amazing, acknowledging what she loves about herself and recognizing what she has to offer the world beyond her looks… What I said next didn't shock her at all. I paused, took a deep breath, trusted my feelings and said the right thing at that moment, and slowly, with confidence, I told her…

"*You could wake up looking like a unicorn or wake up looking like a seahorse. It doesn't matter, you're still the same person.*"

She got it! I watched her soften as the realization sunk in. Wherever you are on your journey, be patient with yourself. We never know how long it may take to undo the beliefs, the stories we've held in our minds for so long… But they can ALWAYS be rewritten.

When you begin to embrace the fact that your value as a human being has nothing to do with how you look, you will become less and less fixated on your appearance or how it is perceived.

When you decide to focus on all the innermost qualities that make you, YOU... That will become what you see. Your truth will shine bright from the inside out as your body's appearance becomes neutral to you and you see what you really are, which is BEAUTIFUL. Period.

While being kind to yourself is the best thing you can do in those situations when the "mirror" just isn't your friend… Find something to focus on that you're grateful for and really feel that gratitude. Gratitude is one of your greatest superpowers, so embrace it! Feeling grateful holds the potential for turning every decision you make, every thought you have, every goal you set for yourself, into a positive one. If your goal is to be healthier and also to make peace with food and your body, you might recite gratitude affirmations such as…

- *I am grateful for the food I have to eat, and that nourishing food is always available to me.*

- *I am grateful for my senses so I can smell, see and taste the food I eat.*

- *I am grateful for my loved ones whom I get to celebrate with, sharing the joys of food and life.*

- *I am grateful that I always have the choice to eat what I want, when I want it.*

- *I am grateful that my body is capable of processing and digesting the food I eat, using it all to energize my body, my mind, and my spirit.*

- *I am grateful for my skin which protects my organs inside and morphs however it needs to keep me safe and healthy.*

- *I am grateful for my strong, powerful legs that carry me through this life.*

- *I am grateful for my big, beautiful bum that helps me sit and rest with comfort when my legs are tired*

Take some time to journal now

Come up with a few affirmations of your own! You can be more serious or have fun with it, but get creative, be specific, and challenge yourself to see how many statements you can write down.

When you are grateful, high vibrational energy runs through your whole body, which makes loving yourself and your life become almost effortless! However, there's more to it than just saying the words. FEEL into your affirmations until you believe them, until they become your reality. When you let yourself get carried away with the power of gratitude flowing through your veins, it can alter your physiology and improve your health.

Thc more specific you are with these the better they will work for you, but it's fine to keep it simple too, especially if affirmations are a new practice for you. Start here…

I am beautiful

I am one of a kind

I am home

That last one for me is all about embodiment… Let's explore this from a literal perspective for a moment.

What makes a house a home?

Some people will say home is not a place, it's a feeling, and I agree. It has less to do with the actual structure of walls and windows, or the color of the paint. It's not about how big or small it is. A house feels like home when you CHOOSE it to be yours. It's a place, an energy, a body that holds space for you, to BE, GROW and LIVE.

So, couldn't you also say that your BODY IS a home? It's the only home you'll *always* have in this lifetime. You were born in it and you'll die in it. The shape and look of your body is not permanent, it's physical appearance WILL change throughout your lifetime and that isn't a problem… That's what makes it so much more beautiful and alive compared to a designed and finished house made of materials or a super-ficially fit body. You are a living, breathing, evolving being that ebbs and flows.

Soak in the truth, let it marinate… The only way to have a body you love is to first and foremost choose to be in the body you have. So, will you CHOOSE to live here in your body and see all the wonderful things that make it unique and feel like home?

There is no one exactly like you, and that is your power. Embrace what makes you special! There's nothing fun or inspiring about going through life trying to be like everyone else. Why waste your time trying to make your body perfect, when perfection doesn't even exist? You don't need to be anything other than your truest, most fully expressed self.

That is beauty. That is confidence. That is self-love.

Here's the thing… you get to live with your body 24/7, so why not do the work it takes to be at home, at peace, and in love with your body NOW? Why not practice unconditional kindness towards yourself? There are so many reasons to be grateful for our bodies. We can feel gratitude simply by acknowledging what our body has done for us in the past, what it does for us now, and we can even feel gratitude for things that haven't happened for our bodies yet.

I submerged my body in a hot, essential oil-infused bath one winter night. I love baths so much and this particular tub time was the first I'd had in over a year! So, I decided to make it special. I had my speakers on the countertop serenading me with relaxing spa music and I even lit a candle. I couldn't wait to just enjoy the moment and feel the warmth on my skin for a while.

I looked down at my belly at one point, half-exposed out of the shallow water. For whatever reason, I started to feel so much positive, loving energy rush all over me as I thought, "This body is brilliant and I'm so grateful it's mine. It's hard to believe this body might carry a baby one day! Woah! I actually have the power to pass down all of my traits into another human being. That is beyond words, amazing."

Happy tears started to dance down my cheeks out of appreciation for my own body. Gratitude allowed me to love my body for something it hasn't even done yet, simply because I knew it was capable. That was a beautiful moment I had with my body, this imperfect and resilient body. The thing that hit me the hardest was realizing I wouldn't have, experienced a feeling like this in the past when my life revolved around controlling the shape of my body instead of loving my body for what it does. When you eat and exercise in spite of your body and speak negatively about it, then feeling any amount of genuine gratitude towards your body will be nearly impossible.

There are an infinite number of ways we can find love and appreciation for our body when we get out of our head and feel for what it needs and craves from us. Usually, it's more kindness and gratitude, but consider what else you might need at this time. What can you give your body more of right now?

Your body loves you. Will you love it back?

Chapter 14

Just Dance

As a gift to one of my clients, I sent her a stainless-steel cuff bracelet engraved with the mantra, "Just Dance".

It was meant to be a daily, loving reminder to choose what makes her feel good, happy, and alive in her body. In one of our previous coaching calls, we started to discuss her current exercise routine and I asked her to tell me what type of movement is the most inspiring, enjoyable, and makes her feel great to be in her body. **She told me she loves to dance**. Shocker! Who doesn't love a good dance session in their living room?? We've all heard the saying, *dance like no one's watching*... That's what **living** looks like.

Movement, exercise, physical activity... I use these

words interchangeably. I've had so many conversations about movement where someone has no problem sharing how frustrated or guilty, they feel about how they "fell off their routine" and they can't seem to get back into it, no matter how badly they want to. I say "no problem" because it seems to me that deep shame around exercise has become very much normalized in our culture today. Just like dieting - it has been a staple conversation in our day-to-day routine for decades. I've watched the industry slowly graduating from this way of living in recent years, but I'm so ready to witness a real shift!

To do my part, I guide my clients through a different way of approaching physical activity. When people tell me it's a "struggle" to move their body... I immediately think, if they *really wanted* to get back into their 'routine', then they would have done it already. Hear me out...

When my clients and I explore what they might have done in the past, it usually comes out in a bland, exhausted tone of voice and they tell me something like:

I joined a gym and dragged myself out of bed at 5:30 AM five days a week for an early morning class before work.

Or

I signed up for a 30-day free trial of hardcore, calorie blasting, at-home workouts that I stopped doing after, well, 30 days…

Or

I had an injury and never found the motivation to get back into it.

The bottom line is **movement shouldn't feel like a chore**. It also shouldn't be something you're either doing at full speed ahead or not at all. Any way that you are able to *move your body* - outside in nature, or indoors in your living room - is just as good for your health and wellbeing as what you would pay for or get at the gym. But any movement that feels like a burden, or is exhausting and unsustainable, or is simply boring and not exciting to you… is actually *not* as good for your health as doing something you honestly enjoy.

So, start there… What do you WANT to do?

Movement is expression. It's meant for so much more than burning fat and losing weight. When you are able to finally realize that fact, I can only imagine what you'll choose to do. You'll probably no longer care for exercise that is just plain old exercise - something that is short-term and is another thing on your to-do list. Instead, when you decide to move your body for the purpose of self-expression, self-reflection, joy, freedom, letting go, relieving stress, healing, strengthening, stretching, connection, and so much more… You might be surprised at what you discover, and that it doesn't even feel like exercise.

While I do teach and practice yoga, my roots are in dance. I started taking lessons when I was three years old and I always loved to perform, but I primarily danced to connect with friends and enjoy myself. It wasn't until my freshman year of high school that I decided to take my dance journey more seriously.

My entire competitive dance career throughout high school and college was driven by superficially admiring my body in the mirror, followed by picking apart my physical reflection, and striving to make my movement appear as perfect as I thought it needed to be in order to feel accepted and good enough - and this extended to other areas of my life, far beyond my dance performance. It later affected how I ate and how I treated myself, which you now know all about.

Liana Blackburn explained this so well in an interview with the founder of Eva Collective for Social Icons where she said, "I see how much dancers are focused on their physical reflection, and not focused enough on their internal reflection." I was never aware I had struggled with this until recently.

As I'm writing this… It's five years after my dance career took a pause, five years after graduating from college and having to step away from the company I co-created and spent most of my undergraduate time and energy developing. This year, I started taking private ballroom dance lessons. Ballroom is a completely foreign style to me, but I immediately realized what made it so special. For me, it offered a new way of looking at dance. Dancing with a partner provides me with a greater sense of connection, elegance, and true self-expression. Dancing belly to belly with only one other person, I don't have to look like or stand out from a whole team of dancers… I only need to be myself.

It's overwhelming at first, having a dozen different styles of traditional dances thrown at you all at once, but my instructor is phenomenal. He intuitively guides me in a way that I've always needed, and he constantly reminds me to embrace the "not knowing" phase of learning something new - which he could probably tell right away is a challenge for me.

In our first lesson, he had me close my eyes at one point, which forced me to fully trust him to lead and FEEL for where he was taking me. I had never done that before. With dance, I was always in control of my own body, and I thought that was confidence. But in those few minutes, I allowed myself to be moved, without knowing what my body looked like. I glided across the floor with his gentle push, and I surrendered into the power of feminine energy - receptive, sensing, flowing.

Contrary to what I believed before learning how to dance with a partner, it was so much better than thinking I needed to be in control. I always imagined I wouldn't enjoy this way of dancing because I would become impatient, and secretly want to be the one to lead the steps. Actually, the *feeling* part of dancing is extremely freeing.

Feeling is living.

This year, having been mostly isolated at home because of the pandemic, I've embraced another way of using dance - for my mental health. Moving the body allows stuck energy to flow through it. Stress, emotion, story, trauma… it all lives in the body. You can use dance, or any way of moving that you like, to uplift or to heal throughout the day. I've noticed on the days where I am spending more time with my clients and doing back-to-back sessions or have long meetings as I sit and stare at a computer screen, movement breaks have been a game-changer!

Exercise doesn't have to be an hour at the gym.

Think of exercise as simply moving your body and consider how you can add more movement throughout each day. Get creative. Think outside the box! Imagine what could happen over time when you just take baby steps…

You could park farther away from your entrance, use the bathroom on a different floor of your house or office building, commit to taking short breaks for movement or stretching, walk away from your desk, invest in a standing desk, spend 10 minutes a day cleaning the house or doing dishes or folding laundry, play outside with your kids, your pets, your friends… The list is limitless!

Take some time to journal now

- *What movement helps you to feel grounded in your body?*

- *What movement helps you to feel at peace and alive?*

- *What do you love doing?*

Maybe it's yoga, walking, stretching, swimming, biking, hula hooping, gardening, playing with your kids, power shopping at the mall, or even getting intimate with your partner? Not sure?

When in doubt, *just dance*!

Chapter 15

Go for Seconds

I had a second piece of cake… and I loved it! No guilt. No shame. I wasn't eating it in secret, and it was NOT a binge! Grabbing another serving from the dessert table was a conscious choice in which I embraced every bite of. The best part was that my decision to eat two pieces of confetti cake with the most decadent cream cheese frosting at 9 pm at a graduation party last weekend, had absolutely no effect on my mood or food choices the next day… My past self would never have even imagined this being possible.

There was a point in my life where I thought I'd always struggle with food… forever analyze it and never be fully okay with my body. I share this to remind my clients (and you) that whatever you are battling now is only temporary. But at the same time, you must first *decide that it will be temporary.* I say that with so much intention, so take a moment to soak in these words… You will only overcome a battle when you decide not to get comfortable in it.

One of my business coaches says, "Choose your hard."

While getting uncomfortable as you work to change your mindset and behavior will probably not be easy… It is just as hard to stay comfortable where you are, even if you are unhappy and know deep down there is a better way. You don't have to change your approach to wellness if you really don't want to, but it's not fair to anyone else or to yourself, especially, if you're going to continue doing what you're doing without seeing the results you want. While letting go of what you know is uncomfortable, imagine what you might discover once you choose to go out on a limb and trust yourself!

While I've already talked plenty about mindset (and I may still weave it in certain places here) I want to dive deeper now into the ACTION of it all and share some of the specific things you can shift in terms of how you're being with food that can make the biggest long-term impact on your overall health and well-being.

This is not a guide on what to eat specifically – I

genuinely do not coach my clients in that way unless it makes sense to because I don't believe it's the most effective way for most people. Here's what I inherently believe... You KNOW what to do with food. From the time we are born we intuitively understand how to nourish our bodies in the right amounts - babies cry when they're hungry, and wean away from the bottle, nipple, or spoon when they're done. You're not broken or uneducated when it comes to nutrition... You've simply lost your way and my goal as an eating psychology coach is to guide you back to your truth. I do my best to enhance my clients' values and add to what they're already doing so that we can move towards even greater success. By shifting their approach even if the slightest, helping them to get unstuck along their journey.

So, let's explore more of that now!

But first, promise me that you will do your best to let go of what you think you know about food and nutrition. Often, in order to learn, we must first unlearn.

So back to my cake story...

If you're thinking, *Lindsey, are you really giving me permission to go for seconds??* Yes, I absolutely am! I intentionally chose to start off this section talking about cake because it allows me to bust a few myths right out of the gate around what it means to eat healthy (for your body, mind and soul), have a body you love, and live a happy life filled with freedom around food.

If you want to feel at peace with food, it's imperative that you get over the fear of overeating.

The most common false belief that our culture has around food is that **we eat too much**. And while that may be true, it may NOT be true for you. Let me rephrase that because this is so important… While America certainly has a problem with over-production and overconsumption of food, society also pushes fear in us from a young age that 'we are what we eat' and that eating too much food (especially the categories labeled "bad" - which ironically are the foods that are produced in the greatest quantities - like sugar, wheat, and dairy) has a direct link to weight gain and disease. What do you imagine this dichotomy would create and trigger in us over time? Exactly… *a fear of food.*

When I work with clients who claim they need to get a handle on their eating so they can lose weight… Often what I discover is that they actually eat a fairly balanced diet and a wide variety of foods. As far as quantity goes, they don't give me much to work with! In other words, from our conversation I usually gather that their primary challenge with food is *not* that they're overeating on a regular basis. It's the FEAR of overeating! It's a fear of not having control of what they consume. It's a fear of gaining weight and growing sick.

I'm sorry to inform you here, these things might still occur in a human being's lifetime for *so many reasons, not related to food.* I'm not saying weight gain or disease are inevitable, and nutrition does play an important role, but eating a perfectly clean diet without fun or pleasure for the sole purpose of having a flawless body and extending your life, is not worth losing sleep over. I think you get where I stand by now.

This fear of food drives a scarcity mentality which leads to the guilt and shame they feel when eating what they declare as being 'too much' or when they indulge in the "wrong/bad/unhealthy" foods they think they just need more "willpower" around. First of all, you do not need more willpower with food… No one does.

Most likely, if you feel that to be true, then what you probably need is to **give yourself more freedom, more forgiveness, and more permission around food**.

As Nelson Mandela once said, "May your choices

reflect your hopes, not your fears."

Overeating can show up in several ways and there are really two types of overeating: physical and psychological. The physical symptoms of having eaten too much can show up as signals from your body such as nausea, fatigue or feeling lethargic, bloating, difficulty breathing, digestive discomfort, etc. The other is psychological, the notion or worry that one has eaten too much. In some cases, a person might hold strongly in their mind that they have overeaten, based on their own perception of what "overeating" means, whether it's measured in calories or types of food or quantities of it, even if they physically feel fine.

So, there you have it… Overeating can show up and cause physical symptoms, or it can be a mindset around food leading you to feel bad after eating. Here's the thing about overeating (or overdoing anything in general). Each person has their own vision of what that looks like. So, comparing your plate to anyone else's, or asking for reassurance from other people, will only pull you farther away from your truth… from having any chance at knowing how to listen to and honor your own body's nutritional needs.

Contributing to the challenge of overeating with self-judgment, shame and blame is not going to make dealing with it any easier! Feeling bad about yourself doesn't solve the problem. **So, what can you do about overeating besides blaming yourself** and feeling guilty about it??

You may have learned different strategies from other people, but here's what I have faith in being some of the most essential things you can do that prevent overeating and improve your relationships with food and yourself when you embrace these practices.

The first is to avoid restricting food… Seriously, stop doing this! Whether you are intentionally eating less or having smaller than usual meals throughout the day… recognize when you're telling yourself this is a good idea or a smart "game plan" for weight loss. Truth be told, this is probably NOT serving you well, and here's why…

You might think it makes sense to eat less (or nothing) so you can "save your calories for later" or make up for overeating in the past. But if you're trying to eat the fewest possible calories, points, or any other way of labeling food with a number, you are fueling a scarcity mentality. This not only fuels chaotic behavior around food, it also puts your body under stress and can hinder your health goals in the long run. When you restrict yourself with amounts or types of food, intentionally or not, your body goes into a stress response. Again, this will have the opposite impact on your health than what you're probably going for.

Your brain thinks in black and white, and it doesn't understand that all you're trying to do is muster up some "willpower" to prevent binge eating that delicious cheesy popcorn! All your brain understands is that there's a lack of [insert trigger food here] in your environment. Then all of a sudden, when you finally come across that food - at a party or at the grocery store or when your partner brings it home without your consent - then your brain drives you to overeat it and store those excess calories as fat so you will be protected in the future, when you might not have access to that food again! Is this making sense?

When you put conditions on food, you give it power. When you remind yourself that you can choose to have something, that it's always available, and that you can enjoy it any time, it loses its power, and you may actually begin to crave it less. This relates back to our survival instinct brain: anything of *lack* suddenly becomes priority, and once it's "allowed" or available again, the blaring lights and sirens go off. You unintentionally put yourself in survival mode as your brain doesn't sense that you're trying to lose weight or avoid gaining it. In fact, your brain only wants to keep you healthy and alive and in abundance of everything you need or desire.

Another way to prevent your scarcity mindset from sounding the alarms every time you walk past an ice cream shop… is to stop viewing foods as good or bad. Food is food. Really, it's just neutral, minding its own business. Food doesn't have any power over you unless you give it that power.

I want to take this opportunity to touch on **binge eating**. Binge eating is like overeating on overdrive. It's a feeling of being completely out of control with food and for some people, they might even 'blackout' or feel entirely numb while it's happening. I used to struggle with this personally. What would often happen is I would find myself binge eating at night, not realizing it was closely related to the calorie deficit that I was intentionally putting myself through during the day to lose weight. Silly, silly me.

I obsessively counted calories and avoided certain macronutrients to achieve the perfect body.

*** Consider if you are severely limiting your carb or fat intake. Why are you doing this? Is it intended to be short term or long term? Please consult a qualified registered dietitian if you have a medical reason for doing so, otherwise, cutting out groups of food is just a fad and can have severe long-term consequences.*

Each day, I was unconsciously putting my body under so much stress that by the evening, I would binge eat. I thought something was wrong with me. But really, my body was just trying to protect me from starving because I wasn't nourishing myself enough. The following day, I would restrict food again to compensate for my behavior, feeling overwhelmed, ashamed, and embarrassed about what I did. Can you see how this easily becomes an endless cycle of doom? Catch yourself if this is happening and stop restricting! If overeating or binge eating does happen, continue the next day like it didn't… Eat variety, eat enough. Nourish your body and mind with plenty of food and kindness towards yourself.

The second practice you can take on to prevent the overwhelming agony of overeating, is to challenge our social-cultural ideas about overeating.

In other words, stop putting conditions on this behavior. Overeating, while it is so frequently judged at times, it's also expected in our culture in certain situations, so you let it happen, simply because it's 'allowed'. Why is that? Do you believe that holidays, for example, are the only times during the year where you can eat a lot of food without being judged for it? Overeating doesn't just occur during the holidays, we know this. But that's when we suddenly become hyper aware of it. The problem in this case is not the act of overeating, it's our social judgment towards it. You might subconsciously believe it's okay to overdo it on a specific occasion like Thanksgiving or New Year's Eve or during a funeral… because everyone else is doing it too or it's simply expected and is considered "okay". But any other time, you tell yourself it's NOT okay… If that's the case, then you better believe you're going to take advantage of those "special" occurrences and overdo it!

Here's another example of this… think about your relationship with candy around Halloween. The judgment might be that it's the only time of year you're allowed to eat candy, when in fact, candy is available to you all year long! If you would just let yourself have something sweet any time of the year, the Reese's cups and Snickers bars probably wouldn't feel so exclusive or special during the month of October or on November first when the leftovers seem to haunt you every time you step into the kitchen… Again, it's a scarcity mentality fueling our subconscious behavior around food.

Bottom line: If you feel guilty or ashamed every time you eat more than you believe is reasonable, you're living in scarcity and judgment, which triggers the stress response, which causes more harm towards your health than just letting yourself overeat once in a while without any attachment towards it.

I have a client who recently shared with me that once she gave herself permission to eat whatever she was craving whenever she wanted it… This person noticed the opposite of what she expected would happen!

We often believe that if we have too much freedom, we will completely go off the rails and splurge in a never-ending buffet of cookies, pizza and chips all day every day. Sure, it could happen once or twice. But honestly, do you really believe that after the third time you would still want that? You would probably get sick of that and crave something else. When we talk about cravings… most people assume that only counts for the "bad" stuff.... the stuff they "shouldn't" have. Unlearn that right now and start listening to your cravings so you can honor them!

You can crave watermelon the same way you crave chocolate. You can crave an organic, grass-fed piece of freshly cooked steak with a side of roasted vegetables the same way you crave a slab of ribs and macaroni and cheese from your local barbecue joint. It's all allowed and it's all necessary.

Create an abundance mentality, and this will make all the difference for you with food. Consider overeating, binge eating, or emotional eating, whatever you may be facing, it's not a 'food' problem. It's a wakeup call from your soul to slow down and explore what else in your life needs attention.

Take some time to journal now

- *Write about the last time you believed you overate.*

- *Were your symptoms of overeating physical, psychological, or both?*

- *What do you believe triggered or contributed to your behavior or feelings of overeating in this experience?*

- *How can you reimagine your relationship with food to prevent this from affecting you in the future?*

Chapter 16

Nature Does Not Hurry

"It's not a 'food' problem. It's a wakeup call from your soul to slow down and explore what else in your life needs attention" - to notice and respect the parts of yourself that need more of your consciousness, your responsiveness, your patience, your love.

When I realized this for myself, I imagined that a heavy hurt I was holding onto was finally lifted. What I once viewed as a time in my life where I was completely failing at something I 'should have' been good at, the truth is that I wasn't failing at all. The way I was being with food (that was taught to me from the world) was failing me. When I once judged myself so hard for losing my mind over a 'binge eating problem' and feeling obsessed about my weight, at the same time I was studying to become a professional nutritionist, I realized that **my real**

challenge, the battle I faced deep in my heart and my soul, was not a problem with food. My perfectionist mindset and deep desire to control were rooted somewhere else. Since health and fitness were important to me, my fears chose to manifest themselves in that area of my life so that I would certainly pay attention! The Universe has a funny way of showing us what we need to see when we refuse to listen otherwise.

This awareness taught me a lot about myself. It caused a great amount of relief, accompanied by a hint of sadness… because I realized my work wasn't finished. While I may have overcome my battle with food and am relieved to know what I know now, my reality is that *perfectionism* and *control* still tend to show up in other areas of my life. For example, I have watched them manifest in my business, especially in the beginning when I first launched my company as a solo entrepreneur. I've watched perfection and unfair expectations, towards myself and others, impact my current relationship, which I see as being the most promising partnership I've had to date and quite frankly, I don't want to screw it up! The point being, the **root cause** of my 'food problem' was not addressed, which is partly why I am so intentional now about helping my clients heal to the core - to work on themselves within a significantly deeper layer than any other diet or nutrition plan could possibly provide… When we know better, we do better.

One thing I know about myself (and see if you can relate to this) is that I tend to put a lot of pressure on myself… Hands up if you know what I mean! Some call that perfectionism, which is why I speak on this topic so much in the book. I'll admit, I was in denial for a while (and I still might be at times) regarding my own perfectionist tendencies. But it really is helpful to identify, not only how it holds us back, but also where it shows up. Perfection mindset is a sneaky one, and it will manifest in more than one place at a time without our conscious awareness.

Bottom line: our challenges with food often go deeper than food. If we avoid or neglect calling them out and holding space for whatever those issues may be, we do ourselves a disservice.

Once I decided to focus less on being perfect with food and more on my well-being, my happiness, my self-confidence from within, and put more of my attention back into what truly mattered… I was able to release my challenging relationship with food naturally, and truly begin to love and appreciate my body again. Looking back, I imagine this being an easy process with flawless execution. But perhaps I'm simply so far removed from this toxic way of being with food that I can't believe that was my life!

The reality is that I couldn't fully recognize or appreciate the incredibly tough journey I went through until years after I found myself in a better place. I don't like to use the word 'recovered' because I don't see any journey we live through as being temporary… I don't believe you are broken until you are healed and then fixed forever. I see this journey as being lifelong, with many twists, turns and opportunities for growth as we continue to learn about ourselves and how we are showing up in the world, as long as we're alive. Some seasons may be more challenging than others, but it is all necessary and each part has something to teach us once we are able to look back on your journey with love. More importantly, practice loving yourself and being okay with where you're at **while you're in it**. That, my friend, is the greatest thing you can do for yourself. In other words, you don't have to wait until you're *there* to appreciate the lessons that are unfolding *here*.

When in doubt, slow down and be present.

Take a moment to pause, to be where you are. It's perfectly okay not to know what your deeper battles are. It's entirely fine not to understand what roads lie ahead. Take it one day at a time, one step at a time, one bite at a time. The greatest practice I've learned, and have shared with each and every one of my clients… Is the power of Slow.

"Nature does not hurry, yet everything is accomplished" - Lao Tzu

Remember this the next time you get caught up in the idea of trying to lose weight, fast… or figure out your overeating problem, fast… or try to heal your gut, fast. Everything in nature happens in the right timing, its own timing. When I work with my clients who wished their challenge with food and body was "fixed a long time ago," I ask them to pause and ask themselves what this challenge might be there to teach them. Yeah, it sucks, and no one deserves to feel the uncertainty and frustration that I felt, the others felt, that you may be feeling now. But the deeper "lesson", if you're willing to acknowledge that now, might be so obvious. Nine times out of ten, an insight will be shared with me that suggests my client needs to **slow down** (and not just with food).

To slow down in life, I help my clients relax around food and take in their eating experience more fully… Breathe. Close your eyes. Say a prayer or a mantra to honor what's in front of you. Say an affirmation to honor your body for being capable of receiving this gift. Before you even take a bite… Look at your food. Notice its colors, textures, size. Smell your food, inhale its aromas. Then taste it… Really taste it! If you enjoy eating with others, who are you eating with and why? If you prefer to eat alone, why? Get curious about your personal eating experiences and notice what contributes to or takes away from making it enjoyable and pleasurable for you. When you eat with others, choose to be with people who lift you up. Engage in positive, light conversation before and while you eat whenever possible. When alone, make it special. Use this time to honor yourself and honor your food by being present with it.

Your true well-being reflects your environment. This includes your external surroundings as well as your internal world. Are you eating in a chaotic environment? Are you rushing through your meals? Are you second guessing your food choices? Are you feeling embarrassed or guilty about what or how much you're eating? It doesn't matter if you eat the purest, most nutritious, most organic, most perfectly balanced meal of all time… The mental, emotional and physical state you find yourself in when you eat (and over time) will powerfully impact your digestion, your calorie burning metabolism, your immunity, your energy, your overall health and well-being.

Slow is the way to go. Slow is about a lot more than just the pace in which you eat… Slow is sensual, it's grounding, it's honoring your preferences, establishing your boundaries, and respecting yourself. Slow requires self-awareness; it encourages making any changes necessary in your external or internal environment so that you can fully appreciate your food, yourself, and the present moment. Slow is nourishing. Slow is comforting. Slow is healing.

We give ourselves more space to listen, to hear what our gut is telling us, and to understand what we need to learn about ourselves when we stop rushing to find the answers… When we stop rushing to "fix the problem" - We open ourselves up to attract what we desire when we stop searching for it. Slowing down helps us to realize our preferences - our likes and dislikes with food. It helps us to get out of our heads and feel using our senses; so, we will stop eating just to check off boxes and eat for the sake of living and nourishing our soul.

We need to get over the fear of slowing down if we ever want to have real, authentic, long-term success and a life we perceive as being abundant in well-being and freedom.

Take some time to journal now

- *Practice slowing down. Start with one meal and see how it goes. Write about what you discover when you do this. What was uncomfortable or challenging? What was easy or enjoyable?*

- *Keep practicing!*

Chapter 17

Have a Smorgasbord

Is there really anything wrong with eating what you want, when you want it? *Never*. Would anyone truly care if you acted on your 'bizarre' craving for pizza AND sushi in the same meal? *Nope*. Is it too much to eat the apple with nut butter AND a bowl of popcorn for a snack? *No way*. Here's the thing: there is no rule (unless you give yourself one) that claims you must decide between meals or snacks and only pick one. Whoever told you that wanting more than you need or desiring multiple types of anything was asking for too much??

I learned this lesson with food a long time ago, and now I'm exploring it in other parts of my world, and it's this:

Let go of thinking that it's wrong or selfish to desire *too much*, ask for *too much*, or believe that you are *too much*. Be ALL that you are, sister, and don't hold yourself back by trying to please others or fit into a certain narrative.

By playing small and not speaking up for what we need out of fear, we risk growing resentful. By approaching our wellness goals in the same way - with hidden perfection, unrealistic expectation, or doubt in our desires - we risk becoming resentful of our health journey. So, when it comes to food, give yourself permission to follow your taste buds, to honor your intuition, to respect your needs… Then watch your confusion, your uncertainty, your hindrance, and your indecisiveness slowly disappear as your confidence in yourself expands.

Growing up, anytime we had multiple leftovers in the fridge, and we needed to eat them up, my mom would call it 'having a Smorgasbord'. I enjoyed these nights! It was a little bit of variety mixed with simplicity as we satisfied our bellies, and my mom didn't have to cook. Win-win for everyone. Now that I'm living in a state of mind where I know I don't have to be perfect with food, I love my smorgasbord meals and snacks! They're usually spontaneous and never followed by shame or regret. In the past, eating more than one thing would have easily felt like 'too much'. But there's a difference between completely losing control with food and making a conscious choice to eat something without second guessing yourself for making that choice! **That's where giving yourself permission comes into practice**.

Many of my clients struggle with feeling indecisive around food - there's just so many options these days, and their perfection mindset triggers anxiety and stress over making the right choice! So, what if you didn't have to choose? Part of giving yourself permission with food involves being flexible. Allowing flexibility and freedom in the way you eat means pulling yourself out of the **all-or-nothing mentality** challenge that most dieters face. We think we need to be all in if we want to have any chance of something 'working' for us... But the truth is that this approach almost always works against us. All-or-nothing keeps us small in our thinking and limited in our success and it stops us in our tracks when we slip up even the slightest! When we let go of trying to be perfect at something, we are more likely to stay present with ourselves on our journey towards better health long-term versus the starting and stopping of diets and plans.

So, what does this have to do with having a smorgasbord, or going to a buffet, or eating multiple things in one meal? It challenges our fear of overdoing it with food by asking us to step into the power of mindful eating and intuitive eating. By having more options to choose from rather than a 'done-for-you' or a 'this-is-all-you-can-have' kind of meal plan… We give ourselves the opportunity to practice slowing down. This way of being with food, along with all the benefits I mentioned earlier, allows us to connect with ourselves on a deeper level to discover what we actually like, enjoy, and want to eat as well as what our bodies are needing us to eat! People think they want the simplest, least complicated path to losing weight or 'knowing what to eat' by subscribing to a pre-made meal plan or a specifically written out diet program… *But no one really wants that*. We want to learn how to eat for our bodies and we want freedom with food! But it does take work and the work is worth it. This kind of effort in learning how to connect with your body is the secret sauce.

You might not believe me when I say that your body talks to you… but it does. We just need to practice slowing down enough to listen. So often, I sense the fear that people have with this - they expect their bodies will only crave junk - better known as their 'fear' foods or 'trigger' foods. I promise you, that's your head talking… not your body. In order to listen for the guidance from your gut you must be willing to trust it. As you work on trusting yourself over time, your natural ability for intuitive eating, and shifting your eating habits with the needs of your body throughout the seasons, will come more easily.

Living in a society where food is available in abundance will feel like a blessing rather than a burden or a confusion, because you'll know what to do - you already know what to do!

By trusting your body and giving yourself unconditional permission to eat without an all-or-nothing mindset driving your goals... Eating will feel more natural, easy, fun and free.

Here's an example of what I mean by "shifting your eating habits with the needs of your body throughout the seasons". No one knows your body better than you do, which is why (now more than ever with the infinite amount of nutritional information you can find these days) it is so incredibly important to listen to your body, your inner nutritional guide – give it a chance!

I talk about "seasons" with my clients a lot. And I'm not referring to eating foods that are 'in season' like summer, fall, winter and spring. I'm talking about your own seasons that you as a unique human being go through. I can identify at least seven seasons that I went through personally over the last twelve months. There was the $3 fast food pizza season, the baking oatmeal cookies and banana bread season, the restaurant quality Home Chef meal kit delivery service season, the buttered noodles and macaroni and cheese season (but let's be honest, we're still in that one), there was the no appetite or taste for anything season, the vegan/vegetarian season, and now on the rise is the cutting down on the types of foods that contain gluten season.

I won't go into the specifics on each of these phases or why they happened for me, but I'll tell you this… NONE of them were about following fad diets, food trends, or giving into laziness (one might assume looking from the outside). Each of these seasons were a genuine shift in balancing what my mind, body, heart and soul desired, or what felt right for me at that time. It could have been what was fun, what was inspiring, what was nostalgic, what was comforting, what I craved, what was healing, or what was necessary. Some seasons lasted several weeks or months, and some for only a few days. The problem I have with the all-too-common all-or-nothing mindset, is that in this space we don't give ourselves enough permission to shift and honor ourselves with as much love as we could. None of my recent food phases were encouraged or inflicted on me by the outside world… ***They came from within***, and I never asked for reassurance from anyone else because I don't need that anymore.

Since Intuitive Eating is my 'lifestyle', I was able to respect my physical, mental and emotional well-being with food in many ways over the last year - the year we faced a global pandemic - the year that was entirely different than any other! I watched so many people try to keep their eating and exercising habits the exact same as before the pandemic started and felt so much shame when they diverted or stopped altogether. When life asks us to step up and be a different person, or focus more on what needs our attention and healing... Our lifestyle habits may need to change or shift for a season and that is okay. It's OKAY.

Okay, maybe it's not the greatest idea to put your body through a seven-course meal every single night... But remember that eating mindfully and intuitively is not about eating perfectly. It's entirely understandable (and sometimes necessary) to honor yourself with the foods you desire, and the foods you crave - even if it doesn't make sense to other people! You're not other people... You're you. So BE you and let yourself eat outside the box.

When and why did we decide that food and nutrition must be so serious? Stay curious with food! Use food as the doorway to explore your sense of self, your values, your desires - on your wellness journey and in life.

Can you achieve an optimal state of health and well-being, even if breakfast looks like a burger on a bun with a side of fresh fruit? Yeah! Or dinner one night is pancakes and bacon with a scoop (or two) of ice cream? Absolutely! Weird? Maybe, but it sounds good to me… that's why I wrote it! Cravings can be strange sometimes, but over the years, I got sick of always trying to be perfect and do it the 'right' way. There's nothing wrong with letting your rebellious teenager come out occasionally and breaking the rules… But it's only breaking the rules if you choose to have them!

If you want to feel at ease with food and exercise TRUST between yourself and your body, stop worrying about getting exactly what you think you need nutritionally every single day. The days of striving to create perfectly proportioned and balanced meals of a protein, veg, carb… Are over. *Wow! Wise words from a 'nutritionist', eh?*

The reality is that food and nutrition are not always a perfect science; humans are not flawless machines with formulas that never change… But we treat our health goals that way and then wonder why it isn't working! Let go of associating any numbers with food - calories, macros, grams, points, servings - and focus on the food! Your body is smart enough to absorb what it needs and use it for energy when it needs it. Think more about what you are getting over time, perhaps over a week, rather than breaking it down and calculating your nutrition day by day, or worse, meal by meal. Eating really does not have to be that mathematical or scientific. Food is nourishment for the body, mind and soul; let's treat it that way. Especially with all the supplements we have available to us these days, please learn to trust that your body is getting what it needs.

If you've made it this far along, you realize now that this book is not a nutrition guide… I honestly feel we have enough of those floating around, and they're ALL going to contain conflicting messages anyway. You can use these guides as resources, as tools, as nuggets of information.

Consider your peace of *mind*, how you feel in your *body*, what you do in the *kitchen*, and start to notice how they're all connected!
At the end of the day… Go with your gut.

Eat what you feel best eating.

Move how you want to move.

Live your life, *perfectly, imperfect.*

About the Author

If you had asked me in college what I would end up doing for work, I might have said something like, "I want to work in an office or with a large company and be well-respected for my credentials. I want to teach people about nutritious eating, share and create 'guilt-free recipes, and inspire unhealthy people to get healthy".

At the time, I had no idea how much personal growth and unlearning I still needed to do. I wouldn't realize until years later that my textbook understanding of health was hardly at all what would make a difference for people, and I had to learn this through my journey first.

Now, I'm proud to say that my "office" is wherever I am. My company is an idea that was built from scratch out of my own heart. The healing I guide my clients through has very little to do with generalized nutrition guidelines - it's about redefining what health means for each person and understanding the relationship we have with ourselves. It's respecting that how we speak, think, and feel about our health journey are essential components of 'getting healthy.'

I like referring to this as a lifelong opportunity to discover our unique path to wellness and well-being while embracing all the twists and turns that show up for us, to teach us along the way.

If it wasn't for the mistakes I made, the false hopes I believed in, the lessons I had to learn, relearn and continue to learn today, I couldn't have written a book like this. I couldn't have the confidence to connect with my clients on a deeper level. I couldn't have the empathy and understanding that makes me so good at supporting others in making peace with food and their bodies.

As a mind-body nutrition expert and eating psychology coach certified through the Institute for the Psychology of Eating, I acknowledge that I'm not the only one who views health from this kind of loving perspective. Many others follow a similar approach in helping their clients reach their goals. But we are still few and far between. So many times, I've given a presentation where the people listening have expressed that NO ONE, not a single health and wellness expert or nutrition coach, has ever permitted them to tackle their goals from such a loving perspective. Yet, it makes sense to them. They get it. The abundance of head nodding and "Mhms" and "Wows" I hear from each group of curious individuals reminds me that what I have to offer is not only what people need… It's what they crave. It's what they've been waiting for. It's what they know in their guts to be true. But they haven't been able to witness it being practiced by most health-conscious folks in our culture.

The world is hungry for more love, and I'm ready to share all the love I can!

If you're looking for more personalized coaching or one on one support, please reach out:

Lindsey Antman

Certified Eating Psychology Coach, Mind Body Nutrition & Food Freedom Expert, Certified Yoga Teacher, Body Positivity / Body Neutrality and Mental Health Advocate

www.mindbodykitchen.org

lindsey@mindbodykitchen.org

Made in United States
Troutdale, OR
11/03/2026

56844506R00106